Better Breastfeeding

RODALE BOOKS

NEW YORK

Better Breastfeeding

A Doctor's Guide to Nursing
Without Pain and Frustration

Linda Dahl, MD

Published in the United States by Rodale Books, an imprint of Random House, a division of Penguin Random House LLC, New York.
rodalebooks.com

RODALE and the Plant colophon are registered trademarks of Penguin Random House LLC.

Library of Congress Cataloging-in-Publication Data
Names: Dahl, Linda, author.
Title: Better breastfeeding / Dr. Linda Dahl.
Description: New York : Rodale Books, [2022] | Includes bibliographical references and index.
Identifiers: LCCN 2021027670 | ISBN 9780593233658 (paperback) | ISBN 9780593233665 (ebook)
Subjects: LCSH: Breastfeeding.
Classification: LCC RJ216 .D24 2022 | DDC 649/.33—dc23

ISBN 978-0-593-23365-8
Ebook ISBN 978-0-593-23366-5

Printed in the United States of America

Editor: Michele Eniclerico
Designer: Jen Valero
Production Editor: Serena Wang
Production Manager: Heather Williamson
Composition: North Market Street Graphics
Copy Editor: Alison Kerr Miller
Indexer: Jay Kreider

10 9 8 7 6 5 4 3 2 1

First Edition

For Jodi

CONTENTS

The Wild West of the Breastfeeding World

Most of the 4 million moms who give birth each year in the United States (and 130 million worldwide) try to breastfeed. Sometimes it happens easily, and when it does, we call it natural. But nature is messy. It's full of accidents and near misses, which is where modern medicine steps in. Take childbirth as an example. It is the second leading cause of death in women of childbearing age worldwide and tenth in the United States. If it weren't for medical interventions, such as C-sections, that number would be a lot higher. Pregnancy is no different. Some women spend years and countless dollars trying to get pregnant. Natural doesn't necessarily mean automatic. As with every other part of the human experience, we are grateful we aren't wholly at the mercy of nature. But for some reason, when it comes to breastfeeding, we are made to believe that nature will make it work every time.

The truth is, the majority of moms need help breastfeeding, and a good portion of those moms fail. Even worse, they are coached, coddled, pushed, and convinced to breastfeed for all the positive outcomes, while the negative impact of trying and failing is entirely ignored. Failed breastfeeding is one of the most terrible things that can happen to a new mom. Not only does it increase her chance of developing postpartum depression, but it can also make it harder for her to bond with her baby. This isn't just unfortunate. It's cruel. I should know, because it happened to me.

I got pregnant at the end of my ear, nose, and throat residency. Although the timing wasn't ideal, my decision to breastfeed was a no-brainer. I knew it was best for my baby, and I prayed it would create a bond between us that would outlast my mere six weeks of leave. I assumed I would have struggles, like finding a decent place to pump in the hospital, and figuring out how to pad my chest so I wouldn't leak during surgical cases. Little did I know, my concerns were focused in the entirely wrong direction.

When my daughter was born, we were off to a good start. She latched on right away and was constantly attached to my full breasts. Although my nipples were sore, she seemed happy enough. By day two, however, the soreness turned into a gnawing pain, which, I was assured, was all part of their toughening-up process. "It hurts even though it's not supposed to hurt," one of the labor and delivery nurses told me.

So I soldiered on, pulling out appropriate idioms to bolster my fading enthusiasm. *No pain, no gain* for the lumpy, plugged ducts that littered my breasts. *If it were easy, anybody could do it* for those endless days turned to nights of nursing every other hour for an hour. *Nothing good comes easy* for pumping and only getting half an ounce of milk. From both breasts.

After two weeks, I checked in with my daughter's pediatrician to make sure what I was going through was normal. I didn't want to complain. I was told that every woman can breastfeed, and I didn't want to be one of those selfish moms who *chose* not to. It just seemed a little extreme.

"She's lost some weight," the pediatrician said, "but that's normal in the first few weeks. Keep feeding her and give her some bottles of formula, just to be safe." Formula? Formula was for quitters. I wasn't a quitter. I just needed more specialized help. So off to a breastfeeding support group I went.

What at first seemed like a meeting of like minds quickly turned into worried competition. The other moms weren't nursing as often. And when they latched on their much fatter babies, I didn't see any bleeding nipples.

Then came the weigh-in.

After nursing for a mere twenty minutes, each baby had taken down a good two to three ounces. Mine had taken a fraction of an ounce.

With a furrowed brow, the lactation consultant handed me the number of a private lactation consultant. She assured me that every woman can nurse, so I should keep trying. But I should also consider supplementing with the liquid enemy to be safe.

The private consultant wasn't much help either. After spending a small fortune, I left with no answers. She was unable to get my daughter to latch on any better than I could, and as it turned out, there was no sense in trying. After only four weeks, my supply had dwindled to nothing. Not even the hospital-grade pump she insisted I rent from her helped. For the next four months, even though I attached myself to it religiously, my supply stayed consistently low, at only two ounces for the whole day.

When I finally gave up, I looked back, wondering where I went wrong. I had asked for help and followed the advice I was given. They were the professionals, right? Even though I was training to be a surgeon, I was still a new mom who didn't know what I was doing. The failure had obviously been my fault. Because every woman can breastfeed.

I wish I could say my story is only my story, but, unfortunately, it is the story of countless women. Every year, nearly four million babies are born in the United States. And although, according to the 2018 CDC Breastfeeding Report Card, 83.2 percent of those moms try to breastfeed, less than half (46.9 percent) are successfully nursing at three months. While the discussion over why these rates are so low could go on for days, numbers and rates don't speak to individual experiences. When it's three a.m. and you're a new mom with bleeding nipples and an insatiable baby, individual experiences are all that matter.

The truth is that 20 to 25 percent of moms can't make breastfeeding work no matter how hard they try. And in today's "breastfeeding-friendly" environment, the pressure for moms to nurse is even more intense. But even as support for breastfeeding grows, the advice given by healthcare practitioners is confusing and often downright wrong. Even though more healthcare practitioners than ever support the idea of breastfeeding, the medical understanding of its pitfalls and failures is stuck in the dark ages. Doctors have no training in breastfeeding, but that doesn't stop them from doling out opinions disguised as facts. And lactation consultants, who often have little to no medical background, have become the experts. In desperation, moms turn to the internet and online chat groups, ending up even more confused and frustrated. If things work out, great. Everyone takes credit. If not, moms are led down an expensive road of pain and suffering, only to wind up at its inevitable dead end. The tragedy is that when they finally give up, they are the ones getting blamed for failure.

There are a lot of books about breastfeeding. So how is this one different? First, nearly all other books come from the outdated, patronizing perspective that every woman can breastfeed if she only tries hard enough. Instead of differentiating between normal and abnormal, they consider all breastfeeding experiences part of a continuum of normal. These books focus on avoiding and overcoming common breastfeeding difficulties without explaining why they happen in the first place. Even with new editions, most are way behind the times. They are part of an outdated paradigm. None discuss tongue tie or the myriad oral restrictions that are currently enjoying an overdiagnostic moment. There is no consensus on what these diagnoses actually mean. None of these books are written by a physician who understands the anatomic and physiologic pitfalls of failed breastfeeding. None of these authors will even admit that some moms won't be able to breastfeed no matter what. Breastfeeding isn't always a choice. For many, it isn't even possible. There is a very fine line between supporting breastfeeding and shaming women who don't or *can't*.

For countless moms, breastfeeding has become a bigger

stress than pregnancy and childbirth. Breast may be best, but not if your baby can't get your milk out. How are you supposed to nurse through agonizing pain? Where is your blissful surge of oxytocin? Isn't the whole point of breastfeeding to make it easier to bond with your baby? No one talks about how painful breastfeeding can actually hurt your ability to bond. And if you bring it up, you are called selfish and subjected to the shame police. Just like I was.

When I went into practice, I spent years trying to figure out what had happened to me. Moms and babies often came to the pediatric practice I had been hired into, but instead of ignoring their plight, I listened. I listened as a *mother* first and a doctor second. Their stories were so similar to mine, I knew there had to be an underlying explanation.

What followed was a deep dive into the intricate, complicated process of breastfeeding. I learned about tongue tie and the standard treatment, which involved cauterizing (burning) the baby's mouth to stop the bleeding. I adapted the procedure, performing it more precisely and getting the babies to nurse immediately afterward, avoiding cautery. The results were extraordinary. Babies were able to latch right away. Moms' woes were cured instantly. I was onto something.

My drive to end suffering carried me beyond simple tongue tie and into the uncharted territory of the mechanics of gape and latch. I learned about how the many variables and moving parts have to work both independently and synchronously for breastfeeding to succeed. I studied with practitioners from different perspectives, like Chinese medicine and osteopathy. I learned from seasoned lactation consultants. I studied my patients, recorded my findings, and, after many years, solved an age-old problem. I figured out how breastfeeding works, why it fails, how to fix it–and how to know when it won't work no matter what you try. I developed a new paradigm of breastfeeding.

Word spread about my work, and struggling moms and babies came from near and far because no one else could help them. Over nearly two decades, I have treated more than 22,000 nursing pairs in New York City and the surrounding areas. I am known as the guru of breastfeeding. Some call me a baby whisperer. But I'm just a heartbroken mom who sees myself in every struggling mom, and my daughter in all their babies.

I'm happy to have been able to help so many in my practice. I'm grateful I've been able to teach so many healthcare practitioners through lecturing and my clinical guide. But I want to reach moms directly, bypassing the outdated messages that tell you to try harder and suffer more. You deserve better. Which is why I wrote this book.

Better Breastfeeding is a fact-based overview of how breastfeeding is supposed to work, so you can understand *why* things are or are not working. Only then can you make informed decisions about how far you are willing to go to try to remedy the problems. This may sound scary, but it isn't meant to be. I want you to be fully prepared for every possibility.

This book will empower you with facts instead of placating you with opinions. It will guide you as you walk through the maze of this very complex, sometimes beautiful, sometimes horrible process. It will also protect you from a growing industry of breastfeeding "experts" who are making a killing on failed breastfeeding, creating diagnoses to justify unnecessary procedures. There is a lot of money to be made in failure. And even more money to be made if you think it's your fault.

Better Breastfeeding is what you, a breastfeeding mom, need to know before and during your breastfeeding journey so you can feel empowered in your first act of motherhood, regardless of whether you decide to continue breastfeeding.

NOTE: To avoid he/she confusion, I will alternate between the pronouns "he" and "she" in each chapter. Odd chapters are "he" and even chapters are "she." I understand this may not be all inclusive, but it makes reading the book easier. When it comes to breastfeeding, the sex of your baby doesn't determine outcomes. We are just used to talking about babies in a binary way.

PART ONE

The Basics of Breastfeeding

Breast Is Stressed:

Is Breastfeeding Right for You?

We have long been told that breast is best. This is true for the most part, especially when it comes easily. But, like everything, when something comes easily, we take it for granted. We call it normal. We assume every mom will be able to breastfeed with the same overflow of milk, and that all babies will find their way to the nipple. We hear over and over again that feeding your baby is natural, and nature always provides. Given those circumstances, who wouldn't want to nurse?

The truth is that breastfeeding is no different than anything else. Sometimes it's easy. Sometimes it's hard. There is often a learning curve. And even if you plan on nursing for a long time, you may not make it to the finish line, because not everyone does. We hear all about the benefits: nutrition, immunity, bonding—the list is endless. But what we don't hear often enough is that for some of the millions of moms who give birth each year, breastfeeding is impossible for very real biological and physiological reasons. For others, it is at best uncomfortable and at worst incredibly painful. For still others, it is undesirable for any of a whole host of reasons, from family structure to time management to postpartum complications. Breastfeeding, like childbirth, is not one size fits all. What works for most moms isn't necessarily going to work for you.

Educating yourself before you start breastfeeding is important. Despite what the media, doctors, and family and friends tell you, answers to breastfeeding problems aren't always obvious. If you wait to find help until after you give birth, you could end up caught in the maze of other people's opinions. And trust me, those opinions won't save you when it's two o'clock in the morning and your baby can't latch on to your traumatized nipples. Or when you've nursed for hours and he's still hungry. Although breastfeeding is one of the most beautiful experiences for a new mom when it works, it can also be one of the most heartbreaking when it doesn't. And that heartbreak can linger for months and years after you stop.

While it is wonderful to hope for the best, it's also important to prepare for reality. Your decision to breastfeed is yours and yours alone, and I want to help empower you with the facts before you even start.

The History of Breastfeeding in Medicine

Speaking of facts, why are they so hard to find? Like so much of medicine that pertains to the feminine, there is little medical information about breastfeeding that's accurate. There is no accepted range of normal in our medical textbooks. No mention of how to keep a good milk supply going on boards exams.

As doctors, we don't even learn how a baby transfers milk out of a breast, even though it's one of the most fascinating biological processes. Instead, even as doctors, we are left with folklore, pseudomedicine, and misinformation. With all this confusion, how do you, as a mom, know who to turn to when you run into trouble? And why is so much of what you hear contradictory and misleading? To understand that riddle, we have to dig into the history of breastfeeding in medicine.

Until the early 1900s, the majority of babies in the United States were born at home with the help of midwives. Midwives encouraged things like immediate skin-to-skin contact and keeping baby and mom together for as long as possible, and, as such, the majority of moms breastfed. Moms who couldn't breastfeed had two options: wet nursing or dry nursing. Wet nursing meant having another mom who was already producing breastmilk (usually from a recent pregnancy) nurse your baby. This was the most popular option and was, at one point, a highly organized profession of women who had recently lost a baby and/or struggled to make ends meet. Dry nursing meant giving your baby solid foods, like ground rice or some other grain, and milk from an animal, like a cow, sheep, or goat.

In 1900, as allopathic medicine was becoming a new profession, medical doctors started getting involved. As doctoring took root, so did the medicalization of childbirth. The all-male doctors—women weren't allowed in medical school—had very different schools of thought from those of midwives. They believed pregnancy was a diseased condition that required as much intervention as possible. Moms were encouraged to give birth in hospitals. They were given drugs and made to undergo procedures that actually *increased* the number of deaths in childbirth for both moms and babies. Babies were even separated from their mothers immediately after being born.

Doctors also had strong opinions about human breastmilk and thought it was bad for babies. Instead, they encouraged moms to use evaporated animal milk. When the babies started developing scurvy and rickets, a "formula," with additives such as cod liver oil and orange juice, was recommended. Doctors even gave out recipes for it. Ironically, although these early concoctions were thought to be healthier, formula-fed babies still suffered far more bacterial infections than their breastfed friends. But as the medical profession grew stronger, so did the influence of doctors and their flawed advice.

The industrialization of feeding babies had a similar course. The rubber nipple was invented by Elijah Pratt in 1845. Shortly afterward, the first commercially available formula was produced in 1867 by Justus von Liebig. Similac (which stands for "similar to lactation") was invented by Alfred Bosworth in the 1920s, and other formulas followed. Even late into the 1930s, evaporated milk continued to be used as an alternative because it was cheap and widely available, and "shown in clinical studies" to be just as good as breastmilk.

With all these other options, it's no surprise that breastfeeding became less popular when women's roles in the workplace shifted. During World War II there was a huge decline in breastfeeding rates in the United States. After the war, more than half of all babies were given some type of formula instead of breastmilk. By the 1950s, that number continued to decline, and only one in five women was breastfeeding.

On October 17, 1956, a group of seven Catholic housewives got together in a Chicago suburb and decided to do something about these low rates. They wanted to save the art of breastfeeding and pass it on to other moms, taking the "You can do it if I can" approach. And boy, had they done it! Between them, they had collectively nursed fifty-five children, with raging success. Pooling together everything they knew, they created notes and journals that eventually became a book. That book, which is still available today, is called *The Womanly Art of Breastfeeding*. Inspired by a shrine in St. Augustine, Florida, that is dedicated to Nuestra Señora de la Leche y Buen Parto (Our Lady of Happy Delivery and Plentiful Milk), they named their group La Leche. And a new era of breastfeeding support was born.

Quickly, La Leche League grew from a local to a national to an international organization, blossoming into the La Leche League International (LLLI) in 1964. Their school of thought differed greatly from what doctors were saying at the time. They pushed to keep moms and babies together, encouraging moms to nurse early and for as long as possible. They also challenged the belief that breastmilk was bad for babies, taking the stance that it was all babies needed for the first six months. But, sadly, La Leche couldn't compete with the doctors who continued telling moms to stop nursing. They also had little ammunition against the aggressive marketing campaigns of formula companies. Despite La Leche's ongoing efforts, by 1975, 75 percent of babies were fed exclusively with commercially made formula.

But La Leche didn't give up. In 1985, a group of La Leche

League leaders decided to legitimize their work and become lactation consultants by founding the International Board of Lactation Consultant Examiners (IBCLE). The LLLI served on the board and donated a big chunk of money. It also created the foundational coursework for boards certification. To be board certified as an IBCLE consultant (IBCLC), in addition to lectures and testing, candidates have to do one thousand hours of lactation-specific work within five years of the exam in a hospital, birth center, or community or private practice, or five hundred hours in an accredited lactation program. Anyone can become a lactation consultant, but many IBCLCs are also healthcare practitioners, such nurses or nurse practitioners, who go through the extra training.

According to the IBCLE website, updated February 22, 2019, there are currently 31,181 IBCLCs worldwide, with more than half in the United States alone. California, Texas, and New York have the highest numbers of IBCLCs per state. But despite the lactation community's best efforts, moms still aren't getting the kind of help they need. The United States ranks only twenty-sixth in breastfeeding initiation rates among industrialized countries, leaving it in the bottom three.

Part of the problem is that not all lactation consultants are created equal. Board certification is voluntary, and not everyone who works as a lactation consultant is trained the same way. Furthermore, only a few states have licensing boards to oversee the accountability and consistency of how lactation consultants practice. (For context, consider that manicurists and massage therapists must be licensed to work. If there is no license, they can't lose their license for not following protocols, because there are no protocols.) It also means that most insurance plans don't cover their fees, which makes them affordable only for the privileged few.

Another problem is that there are many people who give breastfeeding advice but have little to no training. There are plenty of people to "help," from lactation counselors to doulas and midwives to labor and delivery room nurses, but they usually give you their own version of what works. It's no wonder you're confused.

Which brings me back to doctors. Even with the limitations in lactation support, at least it's something. Unfortunately, you can't rely on your doctors to have a wealth of advice about breastfeeding. How could they? It's not part of their medical training. Even if you ask your doctor, which one would you ask?

Obstetricians seem like an obvious choice. They learn all about female reproductive organs, so they should be able to handle breast pain and nipple damage, right? Wrong. Obstetricians are the first to admit they know nothing about breastfeeding. They know everything there is to know about pregnancy and childbirth and even non-lactating breasts. But once those mammaries change into milk-making factories, obstetricians throw up their hands.

What about pediatricians? In terms of the baby, they take over where the obstetricians leave off. They are very good at tracking milestones and screening for congenital problems, but the specialty of pediatrics is for treating children, not adults. When it comes to breastfeeding, they are primarily concerned with one thing: whether your baby is gaining weight. They rarely ask about the experience of feeding—the late nights, spitting up, or endless crying. If you bring up those problems, they may offer advice for the baby, but not for you. They weren't taught how breastfeeding works, so they can't diagnose when something is wrong. Many just employ or refer to lactation consultants. Even more astoundingly, some doctors will call breastfeeding magical, as if unicorns and glitter explode out of your breasts into your baby's eager mouth.

Some doctors do take a special interest in breastfeeding, but breastfeeding medicine is only a loose configuration of different specialties and healthcare practitioners. Although an Academy of Breastfeeding Medicine exists, it doesn't include nurse practitioners, lactation consultants, and anyone who isn't a doctor. That means professionals who work most often with breastfeeding mothers are excluded, leaving out a big piece of the puzzle. There is no consensus of what constitutes a breastfeeding "expert." There is also no fellowship in breastfeeding medicine. Some doctors who work with breastfeeding moms also train as IBCLCs, but even they can't define the difference between normal and abnormal breastfeeding. Along these lines, I'm not proclaiming myself the world's expert. But I do have a tremendous amount of experience, starting at a time when no one in the medical field wanted to get near this population. As an ear, nose, and throat doctor, I am well versed in head and neck anatomy and how all the parts work together. I am also a surgeon, so I understand how form affects function. My specialty includes patients of all ages, from newborns to the elderly and everything in between—even pregnant moms. When I first started to treat newborns, my colleagues thought

I was crazy. Now the procedures I pioneered are becoming mainstream, even if the understanding behind them isn't.

Even though the medical world is caught in a web of confusion, you don't have to be. With this book I will share what I've learned about the beautiful intricacies and potential challenges of breastfeeding so you can be prepared for what's to come. Armed with the facts, you can be your own best advocate. You can decide for yourself when to push through, when to ask for help, and, if needed, when to throw in the towel.

Breastfeeding: The Full Scope

There are many benefits to breastfeeding, but too often we only hear one side of the story. And while it's great to be aware of all the good stuff, it's also good to see the whole picture. We are fed sugarcoated ideas of what it's supposed to be like, then guilted into doing "what's best" for our babies when the shit hits the fan. Keep in mind that even in the best of circumstances, everything has its challenges. If you run into trouble, don't immediately blame yourself or assume you're doing something wrong. If you understand why something isn't working, you have a better chance of fixing the problem. At the very least, you can make an educated decision about what path you want to take. Here are some unvarnished truths about breastfeeding:

1. *Breastfeeding is natural, but the majority of moms need help.*

    Even though childbirth is natural, no one expects you to give birth on your own. So why should breastfeeding be any different? Although there are a lot of reflexes involved, breastfeeding isn't automatic. You still need to learn how things fit together. Don't be afraid to ask for help. Help can come in many forms, and sources may contradict one another. But, at the very least, a support network will help you see you're not alone. For most moms, free or low-cost breastfeeding groups are good enough to get started. If you're really struggling, you may choose to hire a lactation consultant to come to your home. Sometimes, despite all the help, breastfeeding is impossible. Some moms can't make enough breastmilk. Nearly 20 percent of babies won't be able to breastfeed because of their anatomy. Surgical interventions are an option, but you may not want to go that route. Regardless of your circumstances, don't be afraid to ask questions early and often. Who knows? You may end up teaching your doctors and lactation consultants a thing or two.

2. *Breastmilk is free, but breastfeeding is not.*

Feeding your baby from your breast is convenient for a lot of reasons. You don't have to buy all that formula, for one thing. You also don't need bottled water for mixing, something to heat it with, storage containers, etc. The ready-to-go, pre-warmed milk comes out of you on demand, anytime, anywhere. But even though the milk your body makes is free, the whole process of breastfeeding isn't.

For starters, you need a way to get the milk out besides your baby. Some days you may want to do other things, like shower or sleep, so you can't be his only food source. Or your supply may be an issue. You may have to empty your breasts more often to help build it up, or drain off the overflow to prevent engorgement. To do this, you need a breast pump. Sometimes a simple hand pump will do the trick, but you may want to invest in a personal electric one or rent one of those high-powered machines from a hospital. Breast pumps also come with their own set of supplies, like flanges, and bags and bottles to collect and store your milk.

Lactating breasts have a mind of their own, so you have to be prepared with breast pads and shields. Things that used to trigger an internal response, like hearing a baby cry or watching an emotional TV commercial, may now inspire your breasts give off a liquid reminder that you're a mom. Not only can pads and shields help avoid embarrassing leakage, but they can also protect your nipples from chafing or give them a soft landing place if they are damaged from nursing or pumping. You can even buy milk collectors for when your opposite breast decides to let loose while you nurse.

You may want to invest in a new wardrobe that's designed for nursing. If you depend on your pre-nursing attire, you may find yourself topless or practically naked when you need access. Nursing bras and tops have escape hatches so you can offer up your lactiferous ladies covertly. There are also wraps to help you strap your babies on that can double as a modesty cover. Buttons up the front are great for pumping, especially at work.

To manage the pitfalls of nursing, you may also need products and props. There is a wide assortment of nursing pillows and platforms for every situation. If you develop nipple trauma, you may need special creams or ointments. Engorgement and/or mastitis can require doctors' visits and medications. If you don't produce enough milk, you may still need to buy formula. If you are struggling or just want support, you may need to visit a breastfeeding group, which may have a small cost, or hire a private lactation consultant, which may have a much bigger cost.

3. *Breastfeeding is convenient, but only if you can do it, and it takes time.*

If you make around 30 ounces a day, that means you will feed your baby over 42 gallons of breastmilk over the first six months. Although there is wide variability based on milk supply and flow, on average, expect to spend at least 510 hours (or 21.25 days) nursing over the first six months. The time spent per month can be broken down this way:

a. First month: 30 minutes, 8 times a day = 120 hours

b. Months 2 to 4: 30 minutes, 6 times a day = 270 hours

c. Months 5 to 6: 20 minutes, 6 times a day = 120 hours

Sometimes your baby will be so connected to you through breastfeeding that he won't take bottles from you or anyone else. This can make sleeping through the night a distant memory, and prevent you from getting the bed to yourself. Co-sleeping may end up being the only way to get sleep, so forget about intimacy with your partner. You may have to sneak out of your bed or schedule nonsleeping time for that.

Breastfeeding also makes it hard to go out without your baby, unless you are prepared to pump. Your life will have to be compartmentalized into two- to three-hour slots. Eventually, you'll get used to it, but at first you may feel completely tied to either your baby or a pump. If you have other small children or little help at home, it can be challenging to keep up with your other life duties.

4. *Breastmilk is the perfect food for your baby, but what you eat goes right into the breastmilk.*

Your body creates breastmilk from what you eat and store. So when it comes to breastfeeding, your baby has first dibs. When you take prenatal vitamins and eat more food, it's to help your body replace what it loses through breastmilk. Did you know you need to replace some vitamins, like vitamin D, right away or you can wind up deficient? Vitamin deficiencies are no joke. They can cause fatigue, depression, and low energy and make your immune system less effective.

Your baby may also react to foods you eat that come through the breastmilk. You may have to avoid certain foods, in addition to the obvious no-nos like alcohol and caffeine. Things like dairy allergies, celiac disease, and wheat sensitivities can show up as colic, rashes, and gas in your baby. Some moms have to cut out their favorite foods or go through elimination diets to find the culprit.

If you're taking medication, you should decide with your doctor whether it's safe for your baby. If it isn't, you have to decide whether it's safe for you to stop your medication. Sometimes you must put your medical needs before your desire to nurse.

5. *Breastfeeding is one of the best ways to bond with your baby, but if you struggle and fail, it can be more damaging to your relationship than not nursing at all.*

The primary way you bond with your baby is through the hormone oxytocin. Oxytocin is also called the love hormone. It is released in you when your baby cries, and in both of you when you have skin-to-skin contact, or when you breastfeed *without* pain. If you have a little pain in the beginning, that's fine. But anything more than that sends the wrong signals to your brain, preventing oxytocin release, which ultimately gets in the way of bonding.

Stress and lack of sleep can also wear you out. If your baby can't easily pull milk out of your breasts, you may end up spending all your time trying to mimic nursing. This is not the same as normal nursing for you or your baby, so neither of you will get the same benefits.

6. *Breastfeeding may help you get your pre-baby body back, but sometimes it makes it harder.*

Not everyone has the same metabolism. Not all women lose weight with breastfeeding. Some women burn through calories when their bodies make milk, and some, around 20 percent, maintain or actually gain weight. Breastfeeding isn't the most effective way to lose baby weight, if that's your goal. Some women need to eat more than they can burn off just to make enough milk.

7. *Your breasts get bigger when they are full of milk, but your nipples may also permanently change shape, and your breast tissue could shrivel away when you are done nursing.*

When babies latch on to the breast, they use a tremendous amount of force to extract the milk. Although it should never be painful if the baby is latched on correctly, the constant compression and suction changes your areolae and nipples over time so they fit into your baby's hard palate. Nursing for months or years can lengthen and compress them, permanently changing their shape.

The size of your breasts can fluctuate as well, and the change isn't always temporary. When your breast tissue changes to milk-making tissue, it develops new structures that make and store milk, so your breasts grow bigger. But once you stop producing milk, those new structures go away and turn back into regular breast tissue. Without the hormones driving milk production, sometimes you lose more breast tissue than you started out with. Your breasts may thin out and become saggy and droopy.

8. *Breastfeeding is beautiful, but no one wants to see you do it in public or for too long.*

Yes, breast is best. And there is a huge push to get moms breastfeeding. But when you do it in public, people get uncomfortable. For some reason, exposed female nipples are considered obscene in this country, even when you are just feeding your baby. We could go into a whole discussion about why this is true, but suffice it to say that encouraging breastfeeding but shaming moms who do it in public or for "too long" is an unfair contradiction. Breastfeeding is nothing to be ashamed of. If someone else is uncomfortable watching you do it, they should stop watching you and mind their own business. Even if your child is old enough to ask for your breast. Even if you are breastfeeding more than one child at a time. You shouldn't have to hide away in a bathroom or storage closet to do it.

9. *Breastfeeding should come easily, but when it doesn't, everyone acts like it's your fault.*

Hidden beneath encouraging phrases about breastfeeding is the unspoken assumption that the only reason it fails is because you did something wrong. Even if you follow all the advice and the advice contradicts itself. Even if your breasts don't make milk, or you were taken down the wrong road. At the end of the day everyone assumes breastfeeding failed because you failed. As women, we are conditioned to accept this kind of blame. We are even prepped for it when we are told mistruths about nursing through pain or made to believe every woman makes enough milk. And, for some reason, we embrace that martyrdom. We want to suffer for our children. Giving birth is the ultimate sacrifice as well as the ultimate gift. But breastfeeding should be the opposite. It is the reward you get for carrying your baby and giving birth. It should not be another source of suffering.

The truth is, most of the time, the baby's anatomy is the

reason breastfeeding fails. We will talk about this more in subsequent chapters. That's why arming yourself with medical and anatomic facts can validate your efforts, even if nursing doesn't work out for you and your baby.

10. Even if you are a new mom, you still have the best sense of what is happening with your baby.

Moms hear all the time that we have intuition. Then we show up at a doctor's office with that same intuition and are told that we think too much or are worried about nothing. Even though this may be your first baby, you still have the best sense of what is happening with him. Doctors and healthcare practitioners like to fit things into boxes, and when something doesn't fit, they either brush it aside or assume you are missing something. Even if you can't pinpoint the problem, if you feel something isn't working the way it should, you're probably right. I wish I could tell you that finding the answer was just about asking for more help. It's really about advocating for yourself and researching until you find the answers that make the most sense for you.

2

Milking It:
Getting Ready to Nurse

Now that you've made a conscious decision to breastfeed, let's get ready to nurse! How and what you do to prepare depends on your resources and circumstances. Income also matters, unfortunately. Some help is free or covered by insurance, but some costs a pretty penny. Regardless, there is a lot of help these days for every income bracket and location, especially because there is so much help online. In this chapter, I will walk you through everything you need to do to prepare for breastfeeding *before* the baby arrives. We touched on some of these things in Chapter 1, but I will go more in depth here about things like which classes to take, the supplies you'll need, and where and how to find breastfeeding support. We will talk about the kind of foods to eat or avoid, and questions to ask your obstetrician about how the delivery impacts breastfeeding. If you're a first-time mom, you will also have to think about finding a pediatrician. I'll guide you through that process, as well as how to find and vet a lactation consultant.

Whatever you do, make sure to assemble a support group

before problems arise. Don't try to go it alone. If you wait until you run into problems, you will be stuck looking for help in a desperate state—and desperate moms are easy targets.

Classes to take

Google "breastfeeding classes" and you will likely end up with a whole slew of options. How do you know which ones to choose? In-person classes differ in many ways, but they basically boil down to three categories: those run by La Leche League leaders, those run by private lactation consultants, and those that are part of broader childbirth classes.

La Leche League classes and those run by lactation consultants are primarily meant for post-baby moms, but there is no reason you can't go before you give birth. In fact, they encourage it. Seeing firsthand what moms actually struggle with when they first start nursing can give you the kind of insight you need before you have your baby. I encourage you to go to more than one class and meet with more than one instructor. You will find that everyone has their own style and opinion. Moms also have very different needs. You'll probably learn just as much from the other moms as you will from the instructors, so you can start building your community. The costs will also differ. Most La Leche classes are free, but those run by lactation consultants or counselors usually come with a fee.

There are also prenatal classes presented by those in the "childbirth world," such as prospective pediatricians, doulas, midwives, psychologists, and self-proclaimed experts. Usually, their focus is on childbirth and caring for your baby in the first few weeks, with a lecture here and there about breastfeeding. With all you need to learn, it's not surprising that breastfeeding takes a back seat. But you need more than encouragement and reasons to breastfeed to be prepared for what lies ahead. To succeed, you need to really delve into the meat of things.

More thorough programs that you can attend from anywhere are available online. My favorite was created by my colleague Jack Newman: https://ibconline.ca/online-prenatal -class/. Based in Canada, Dr. Newman has been working with nursing moms for close to forty years. There is a fee, and the classes take a considerable amount of time, but if you can fit it into your schedule, it's worth it. Other, more static classes may give you information, but there's nothing like the emotional connection of immediate need to really solidify what you're learning.

Supplies for Breastfeeding

As I mentioned, breastmilk may be free, but all the things you need to breastfeed are not. There are so many products on the market, I've divided them into categories. Some things are essential, but others are just for fun. Some I hope you'll never need, but I'll explain them anyway so you know what they are.

1. *Breast pump and pump supplies*

Breast pumps are essential. Even if you think you will want to nurse all the time, chances are, you'll still want to do things like sleep and shower. You may even want to visit friends or go back to work. Whatever the case, unless you plan to be with your baby 24/7, you're going to need a way to get the milk out of your breasts that isn't your baby, as well as a way to get your milk into your baby that isn't you.

There are three categories of breast pumps: hospital-grade, electric, and hand pumps. Hospital-grade pumps have the strongest suction, but they are far too expensive to purchase outright. Luckily, with recent healthcare reforms, most insurance plans will cover rentals. Your workplace may even supply them. In addition to hospitals, there are many other suppliers, like stores that carry baby goods, pediatricians' offices, and lactation consultants. You may not need a hospital-grade pump for long-term nursing, but it doesn't hurt to start with one while you are figuring things out. Hospital-grade pumps also give you the best chance at emptying your breasts so you can maximize your supply early on. There may be a delay in getting the prescription for the rental approved, so you should have another option while you wait.

Electric pumps are less expensive, but they aren't covered by insurance. You can purchase one outright and use it for the duration of nursing because you don't have to return it. You can even use it for other children down the road or keep it as a backup for the hospital-grade pump. I don't recommend a particular style or brand because everyone has their own needs, and new styles are developed regularly. Find one that works best for you.

Factors to consider when choosing a hospital-grade or

electric pump are suction power, flange options, ergonomics, double pumping (the ability to pump both sides at once), battery life, and insulated compartments for milk storage. Some are quieter and more discreet than others, but they all require a private place to sit and pump.

Hand pumps are small, cheap, and easy and, for some women, more effective than the motor-powered ones. You may get exhausted trying to manually get all your milk out, but often your body will help you by releasing hormones that push out the milk. There are also simple silicone bulbs that attach to your breasts and collect your letdown. If you are nursing on one side and tend to drip out the other, these collectors are a good way to save your milk and prevent a mess. More on breast pumps and their use in Chapter 11.

2. *Breast covers, pads, shells, silver cups, and shields*

When you breastfeed, your breasts transform from pleasant but useless appendages to milk-making factories. Once the hormones turn on, you have no control over when and where they decide to let loose. Leakage can happen because of something as simple as hearing your baby–or any baby, for that matter–cry, or it can happen for a more obvious reason, like engorgement from waiting too long to pump or nurse. Before you leave the house, it's best to pad yourself with something to soak up the overflow.

Disposable pads are convenient and absorbent, much like diapers. If you want to do your part to reduce landfill, you may opt for the reusable cloth variety. There are also silicone shells that have a dual purpose: They protect your nipples and collect excess milk so you can save it and pour it into a bottle. They are reusable, so they need to be washed regularly.

Speaking of protecting your nipples, if you need the following products, something isn't going as it should. The first is a silver nipple cup. Popular in Australia, these "healing cups" can be filled with breastmilk, then placed over damaged or chafed nipples. Silver is believed to have natural antibacterial properties to heal and protect your nipples when you aren't breastfeeding.

For protection during breastfeeding, there are nipple shields. These silicone areola covers look like hats and have holes in the top to allow milk to come through. They come in an assortment of shapes and sizes, and fit is important. You may first be introduced to them when you start nursing as a remedy for sore nipples. Ironically, if you need them, it likely means your baby isn't latching on deeply enough (more on this in Chapter 9). However, if you need something to tide you over while you sort out the cause of your pain, or if your baby can't latch on at all, these are a good Band-Aid. Keep in mind that they don't fix your baby's latch or help her drain your breasts. They just offer an extra layer of protection from the friction of a shallow latch. You will still have to fix the underlying problem if you want to nurse successfully or long term. Once the underlying problem is fixed, you can use nipple shields to protect your nipples as they heal. Nipple shields can also help a baby who has nipple aversion wean back onto the breast (see Chapter 13 for more on nipple shields).

3. *Pillows*

It used to be that the traditional way to nurse your baby was holding her in your arms, but all that changed with the Boppy pillow. Shaped like an overarching letter C, it's supposed to fit around your waist to cradle your baby in a cross-cradle position while you nurse. The truth is, it doesn't actually fit around any regular human. It works best if it's propped up to chest height by placing a regular pillow underneath it. You can also use it to prop up other parts of you, like to support your bum and protect your post-delivery parts.

Most moms prefer the My Brest Friend pillow. It is much larger and straps around your waist to provide a higher platform for your baby. Because it's hands-free, it is less likely to shift. It also cradles your baby closer to your breast, where you need her. Because of its size, it's harder to lug around, but you will mostly need it in the early stages when your baby is small and you're not traveling as much.

There are other pillows of varying shapes and sizes and some made with materials like memory foam or beads. There is the Butterfly Pillow, which has layers of pillows so you can adjust the height. There is also a Littlebeam pillow, which can be stacked on top of a Boppy or regular pillow. Most have washable covers and double as support for other parts of your body. You can always just use regular pillows. You will need some sort of support early on, but less so as your baby gets bigger.

4. Ointments and salves

In the best of worlds, you won't need anything more than some lanolin or coconut oil to coat your areolae and nipples. But if you and your baby don't have a great fit or if your nipples are sensitive, you may need something more heavy-duty. Medicated ointments are helpful for damaged nipples, especially to prevent or treat infections. Some are over the counter, like Neosporin for bacterial infections or Monistat for fungal infections. But if you have more serious damage, a doctor or midwife may prescribe something called APNO (all-purpose nipple ointment). APNO is a combination of an antibiotic, an antifungal, and a steroid, and has to be made in a compounding pharmacy. Like any medication, it must be thoroughly wiped off your areola and nipples before your baby can nurse. And, like nipple shields, if you need this ointment, check your baby's latch. The damage is most likely from friction and a shallow latch.

5. Supplements

Basic supplements, like prenatal vitamins, are a necessity, not just during pregnancy but also while nursing. Your baby gets everything she needs from you through breastmilk for the first six months, so the vitamins aren't for her. They're for you. They replace what your body loses through breastmilk. Extra vitamin D in particular is important from the beginning for those who live in colder climates, but every mom should supplement after the first six months.

If you have concerns about your supply, you may want to consider taking over-the-counter supplements. Most are plant-based estrogens and have been used by women for centuries. Although there are many brand names, most milk-promoting supplements contain one or more of the following ingredients: fenugreek, galega (goat's rue), silymarin, shatavari, and torbangun. If you're looking for studies that prove that they work, good luck finding them. It's hard enough to measure milk production among women on its own, let alone comparing whether supply increases with supplements. You can follow the recommended doses on the bottles, but avoid taking any of them if you have thyroid disease or other conditions (see Chapter 11 for more on supplements).

6. *A new wardrobe*

Today's nursing tops and bras are comfier and more convenient than their cousins from the past. The biggest difference between nursing-wear and your normal clothes is that they open in the front or have escape hatches that allow you to slip a breast out when you need to. This is especially important when it comes to dresses. Gaining access to your top when you're wearing a non-maternity dress may mean taking the whole thing off.

If you don't want all new clothes, your wrap tops, button fronts, and open V-necks make access easier. There are also wraps with which you can strap your babies on and carry them around that can double as a modesty cover when you nurse.

Food and Drugs to Consume or Avoid

When you breastfeed, you have to think about your diet in ways you probably haven't before. Like in pregnancy, certain foods are off-limits because they are obviously bad for your baby. But there are others that can have an impact on your milk supply—some can increase it and others can wipe it out. You also have to eat more to make up for that extra 30 percent of your daily calories your body needs to make milk. That's even more daily calories than your brain needs, but not quite as much as what you need in your third trimester. But there are a lot of myths about what does and doesn't affect your supply, so let's clear that up first.

Despite what you hear, what you eat changes the nutritional makeup of your milk only a little bit. This includes drinking more water. Although you should stay hydrated, more water doesn't increase your supply, because your supply is hormonally regulated (see Chapter 3). Even if you eat a steady diet of bread and cheese, your body will still make milk that's nutritionally complete for your baby, but it will do it at your own expense. But there are exceptions, and they are important ones.

Vitamins help your baby's development in a lot of ways, so make sure you keep taking your prenatal vitamins for as long as you continue nursing. This not only helps your baby, but also prevents your body from losing its own stores in breast milk production. Prenatal vitamins should include folic acid, iron, calcium, vitamin D, vitamin C, vitamin A, vitamin E,

B vitamins, zinc, iodine, and choline.[1] They should also be free of preservatives and fillers.

Fatty acids are particularly sensitive to what you eat, and they are important for your baby's brain development. The most important ones are docosahexaenoic acid, or DHA, and arachidonic acid, or ARA. You can take them as a supplement (omega 3 fatty acids) or eat more fish. Be careful of large fish, like mackerel or swordfish, because they can also have mercury, which leaks into breastmilk. Fish such as salmon, tilapia, and cod have lower mercury levels, and sushi is okay once in a while.

What you drink matters too. Caffeine in coffee or tea isn't great for your baby. Even though only 1 percent of what you drink gets to your baby through breastmilk, that still may be enough to make your baby fussy or have trouble sleeping. The same goes for alcohol. Even though things like beer and wine have been thought to help with letdown and supply, it's really the plant parts of those drinks, such as hops and barley, that help—not the alcohol. Alcohol can take a couple of hours to break down, and it's obviously bad for your baby. If you want to have a drink, do it after you've nursed to give your body time to get it out of your bloodstream. If you drink enough to feel drunk, it's best to pump and dump it out so you don't pass it on to your baby.

There are some foods that have surprisingly weird effects. Some are thought to cause your baby to have gas, like beans, broccoli, cauliflower, Brussels sprouts, onions, and cabbage. Some, like spices such as ginger and garlic, can flavor your milk in way your baby may not appreciate. Chocolate can act like a baby laxative. And some innocent-seeming herbs, like parsley, sage, oregano, and peppermint, are believed to decrease your supply, while fennel, barley, and oats can increase it. No scientific studies have proven any of these claims, but setting up a study to measure a mom's supply changes is nearly impossible, for whole host of reasons.

It is also possible that your baby may be allergic or have bad reactions to certain foods. If you notice that your baby has a rash, congestion, diarrhea, or gas and/or is fussy, look back at your diet from the six hours prior. The distress may be coming from something you ate. Common culprits are dairy and fruits like pineapple, kiwi, strawberries, prunes, or cherries. Wheat can also be a trigger, especially if your partner or someone in your family has a history of celiac disease.

Drugs to avoid are the same as during pregnancy, but pay particular attention to over-the-counter cold and allergy medications. The drugs in these seemingly innocent preparations, like pseudoephedrine and all antihistamines, can dry up your supply. Sometimes women take them on purpose to stop lactating. Restarting birth control pills or taking steroids for any reason can put a stop to milk production. Before you take anything, or if you notice a sudden decrease in supply, check with your doctor. Prescribed medications may also not be safe for nursing, so talk to your obstetrician and other doctors about weighing the risks and benefits of stopping them. Never do it on your own.

Questions to Ask Your Obstetrician

You will hopefully have a wonderful relationship with your obstetrician during your pregnancy, but most soon-to-be moms don't think about bringing up breastfeeding at prenatal visits. If you mention it to your obstetrician at all, it's usually after the baby comes and only if it isn't going well. It's best to know where your obstetrician stands before you have your baby, so you make sure you're both on the same page. How you give birth can affect your first moments of breastfeeding, especially when your birth method doesn't turn out to be what you had planned.

Immediate skin-to-skin contact promotes oxytocin, bonding, and letdown. C-section births, planned or otherwise, can delay skin-to-skin contact. Postoperative pain medications from the C-section can also get into your breastmilk and make your baby sleepy. If your baby has to go to the NICU, it's good to know the policies regarding breastfeeding. If your baby is premature, her reflexes may not be active enough for her to nurse, or your milk may not come in right away, so they may automatically give her a bottle. It's good to prepare for these possibilities or at least ask about them so you aren't left in the dark.

Some obstetricians work with midwives or doulas who can help you with your birth and breastfeeding plan. They generally have more time and provide more support than the doctor. They may even be able to give you a prescription for a breast pump, so you are ready when the baby comes.

How to Find a Pediatrician

Finding a pediatrician may be easy or hard, depending on where you are and how many choices you have. In smaller towns and less urban areas, you may have only a few options. But in major cities, there are so many doctors that it may be hard to sift through all the options. The best way to start is by compiling a list of recommendations from family, friends, and online groups. You can even check with your insurance plan, local hospital, American Academy of Pediatrics, or online reviews. Start looking at least three months before your baby is born in case she comes early. Then you can get down to the details.

Make sure your pediatrician is board certified, and find out where they have hospital privileges. Some work primarily in hospitals and emergency rooms, whereas others do only private practice. Age may also be a factor. Older doctors have more experience, but younger doctors may have new ideas and be less invested in outdated opinions. If you aren't independently wealthy (and even if you are), it works best if your pediatrician takes your insurance. The size of a group practice will also affect whether you can see your pediatrician every time or see someone different. The bigger the group, the more availability, but you may not always get a consistent message.

Some pediatricians are more breastfeeding-friendly than others. Some are even lactation consultants themselves, or employ them. It is best to meet with a few before deciding on who to use. Don't be afraid to ask specific questions about breastfeeding, like what their recommendations are, how much support they can offer, and how they manage or evaluate breastfeeding problems. Also, see how long they recommend moms breastfeed, when they recommend starting solids, and how they feel about nursing past two years. Ask who they refer moms with breastfeeding issues to, including a list of lactation consultants, craniosacral therapists, and ear, nose, and throat doctors (or dentists) who can do procedures. Whether they are prepared with these lists can tell you a lot about how they view breastfeeding.

Most important, you need to find a pediatrician who listens to you and respects your opinions. Moms really do have intuition. If something doesn't feel right, or if you have a lot of questions, you need to feel heard. It's important to see a pediatrician who is as comfortable with what they *don't* know as what they *do* know. The more consistently your baby sees her pediatrician in the first six months, the more likely she will get all her needed tests and treatments on time, so it would be great to hit it right off the bat. But even if you start out with someone and the relationship isn't what you expected, don't be afraid to switch. Doctors are used to it and don't take it personally.

How to Find a Lactation Consultant

Lactation consultants (LCs) are professionals who are trained to help you nurse, but, like doctors, not all are created equal. Anyone can call herself a lactation consultant, but only some have gone through extra training to become board-certified

IBCLCs. Many others in the childbirth world can help, such as doulas, midwives, lactation counselors, and labor and delivery nurses, but everyone has different training and opinions. Again, it is very hard to know who to trust, because there's little consensus when it comes to breastfeeding advice. What's worse, even if someone is certified or recommended, not every state has a licensing board to keep the narrative consistent between practitioners. Finding someone to help you is a little bit luck and a little bit casting a wide net. You can start your search online through the IBCLC website, through La Leche League, through the United States Lactation Consultant Association, or by asking friends or your pediatrician.

Most moms consider hiring or working with an LC only when they run into trouble. A better plan is to meet with an LC or go to a breastfeeding class before you give birth. That way you can see what moms go through, so you have a sense of what "normal" is. When you run into trouble, it's easy to feel like you're the only one. Seeing other examples of struggling moms can help you be more objective. You can also see how different LCs are in terms of personality and advice. Everyone has their own style. If you rely solely on referrals from friends and others, you may not find someone who is a good fit for you.

Once you have the baby and decide you want to see an LC, you can either make an appointment in their center or attend their classes. If you opt for a private visit, the LC comes to you and spends two to three hours helping you. They often bring a baby scale and supplies, in case you need something like a nipple shield. They can help you figure out your pump and make sure you have well-fitted flanges. They can talk to you about pumping regimen, timing of feeds, and how to read your baby's cues. Essentially, they can give you the lowdown on everything that breastfeeding "should" be. All this attention isn't cheap. It usually costs around three hundred dollars. If the LC is also a midwife or nurse practitioner, she can bill the visit through insurance.

Although most moms are happy with their LCs, I've also read countless online reviews and listened to one horror story after another about what an LC did or did not say or do. This is often the case when you run into more severe or complex issues. Having had the same experience myself, I can understand the frustration from both sides. There is so much misinformation about breastfeeding, including what is reinforced in training programs, that even though everyone is doing their best, sometimes the information they give you is wrong. Sometimes, no matter how hard you try or what you do, breastfeeding just doesn't work. If you are led down the path of "It always works for every woman," and you've spent a small fortune in that belief system, it's normal to feel disappointed. Add to that the hormonal fluctuations of failed nursing, and your anger may even turn into rage. But if you accept the realities of breastfeeding and adjust your expectations, you can make informed decisions so you won't feel like a victim.

However, there are red flags to consider. Any practitioner, LC or otherwise, who tells you "the latch is fine" when you are grimacing in pain is not to be trusted. You can't examine a latch from the outside, because all the moving parts are happening on the inside. You should never just push through the pain, because every moment counts in the first few weeks. If your LC won't listen to you, then, just like with your doctors, find someone else. If things aren't getting better, don't stick with someone who doesn't hear you. You want someone who is in it for the long haul. That three hundred dollars should also include follow up emails and phone calls. And if they refer you to another doctor or dentist for a procedure, ask them why they prefer one over the other and how they can help after the procedure.

The point at which lactation consultants and pediatricians disagree the most is at "diagnosing" the cause of breastfeeding problems. I will get into that discussion in Chapters 9 and 10, but suffice it to say they are using the same language to mean different things. In the end, you may have to be your own diagnostician, but that's okay—this book will provide you the tools to make those decisions.

3

Go with the Flow:
The Mechanics of Breastfeeding

If you consider everything that needs to work for breastfeeding to happen, it's a miracle it works at all. True, there are reflexes and hormones that may make it seem automatic, but there's a lot more to it than that. You and your baby have to come together as a complicated "machine" with lots of moving parts. And just like the delivery, when your baby has to fit through your pelvis, in breastfeeding, your baby's mouth has to fit onto your breasts. Then, your breasts have to respond, pouring out milk when your hormones react to your baby. From the outside, it may seem like a natural coupling of parts, but the real work is happening on the inside—the internal part no one can see. Sadly, that limited outside perspective is what everyone uses to make assumptions about what is happening on the inside. It's no wonder much of what is considered "normal" is highly subjective.

The good news is that there is a solid body of research that explains the mechanics of how breastfeeding is supposed to work when it is working *perfectly*. It is complicated but fascinating, and well worth the effort of learning. It is also rarely understood by those giving advice about breastfeeding.

In this chapter, I will walk you through the mechanics of this "machine," step by step, so you can understand how/when/where/why breakdowns can occur, if they do. Then, if things aren't working correctly, you can have more tools to understand why.

First, let's talk about your baby.

Baby Anatomy

Your baby's head and neck anatomy are very different from yours. His parts are shaped and positioned in a certain way to make breastfeeding possible. In such a tiny package, precision is key. And once you understand all the nuances, you will see why the way he "fits" your breasts is so important.

All babies' jaws are set back a little bit, which makes their chin look smaller than it really is. A newborn's tongue is also larger than an adult's relative to his jaw, and it sits farther back in his throat. His voice box sits in a higher-up position in his throat, near his soft palate (the flexible part of the roof of his mouth that includes that dangly thing in the back). The bridge of his nose is flatter, and his nostrils are wider than an adult's.

Because of these anatomic differences, breathing and eating is different for a baby. With all that anatomy so high up and set back, he is able to breathe only through his nose for the first three to four months. This is actually a good thing, because it allows him to breathe and nurse at the same time. As he is crammed up against your breast, the shape of his nose makes it easier for him to breathe out the sides. His tongue's size and position give it a wider range of motion. And because your baby latched on to your breast is a closed system, when he swallows, milk can go straight down his gullet and not into his trachea and lungs. But because all his parts are so tiny, this system can work right only if everything fits together perfectly.[1]

When your baby gets older, his anatomy actually develops away from being able to nurse. If he isn't nursing as a newborn, he won't suddenly be able to do it when he's six months old.

The Act of Breastfeeding

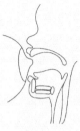

Figure 1: Gape

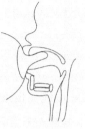

Figure 2: Latch

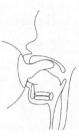

*Figure 3: Suck reflex–
lifting the tongue*

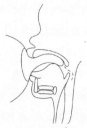

*Figure 4: Suck reflex–
pulling the tongue back*

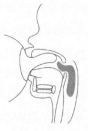

*Figure 5: Jaw drop
and swallow*

NOTE: For simplicity's sake and for purposes of this discussion, we are going to assume here that you have a normal milk supply (not too much or too little), and your baby wants to nurse.

Although everyone focuses mostly on your breasts, pulling out the milk is a two-person process: Your baby must compress and pull milk out of your breast, and your breast has to push it out. We will first talk about your baby's contribution.

You may have been told that the first step in nursing is the latch. But the first step in the latch is the *gape*. The gape is the single most important part of the latch, because without a gape, there is no latch. And without a latch, everything down the road falls apart.

The gape is your baby opening his mouth so wide, he can fit it all the way around the areola, past your nipple, and form a seal. When your newborn gapes, he disengages his jaw, like a snake. Because it is a relatively relaxed position, he should be able to keep his mouth in that position for a long time without getting tired. When the gape happens normally, it allows him to get his mouth around the parts of the breast that have the ducts (tubes that carry the milk), while his tongue, palate, and jaw do the work to get the milk out.

Gaping to latch on is not the same as a regular open mouth for a newborn, or anyone else, for that matter. Babies open their mouths wide to yawn or cry. They may even start out with a wide-open mouth when they go to the breast, then slide down to the nipple once they get on. Neither of these is an example of a normal gape. They are examples of *hinging* at the jaw, but gaping means *unhinging* the jaw.

Another important thing to remember about the gape is that it is a *reflex*.[2] Reflexes are automatic, which means a baby's gape is automatic. When your baby is born, he will automatically gape as wide as he can when he smells your breast. If your baby *doesn't* gape at birth, it means he *can't* gape. It doesn't mean he's lazy. He won't "learn how" or "grow into" it. You can't help him gape by pulling down his jaw or trying to flange out his upper lip. It is a physical unhinging, which means he can either do it or he can't. If he can't, it's an anatomical issue that can be addressed (see Chapter 10 for a discussion of gape restriction).

Once your baby gapes, he is ready to *latch on*. With his wide-open throat, he will be able to get his mouth around all or most of your areola and seal his lips around your breast (*not your nipple*). Your baby's hard palate (or the roof of his mouth) then gets filled with your breast tissue. Your nipple should ideally sit way in the back of his throat, at the opening of his esophagus, where nothing is touching or pressing on it.

When your baby's hard palate is filled with your breast, his second reflex, the *suck reflex,* gets triggered. Interestingly, anything pressing against his palate—e.g., a bottle, a finger, a pacifier—will make your newborn suck. That's because, like the gape, the suck is also a reflex.[3] It's also why when your baby isn't latched on deeply or doesn't have enough breast filling his palate, he may not suck. The same thing can happen with pacifiers and bottle nipples that are too small to press against the roof of his mouth. They can fall out of his mouth, or milk can leak out the sides. The suck reflex starts to develop at thirty-two weeks' gestation and is fully developed by thirty-six weeks.

Once your baby has gaped and latched on correctly, the magic can happen. (When this machine works, it truly is magical, even if there aren't unicorns and glitter.) Your baby presses your areola against the roof of his mouth with his tongue, then pulls his tongue to the back of his throat to compress the milk out. When his tongue goes as far back as it can, he drops his jaw to create a vacuum, which pulls out even more milk. Because your nipple is already sitting over his esophagus, the milk flows out of your nipple straight down the hatch, and your baby swallows. Then the cycle begins again.[4]

Throughout the suck and swallow, your nipple should stay in the back of your baby's throat. It shouldn't move in and out of his mouth or be compressed by his tongue. When your nipple stays where it is supposed to be, it won't be subjected to friction from your baby's tongue, lips, or mouth. No friction on your nipple means no nipple pain for you. This is why breastfeeding with a good latch is not painful (more about nipple pain in Chapter 9).

So far, so good? Let's move on to the other half of the story. Here's a little anatomy lesson about lactating breasts.

Breast Anatomy

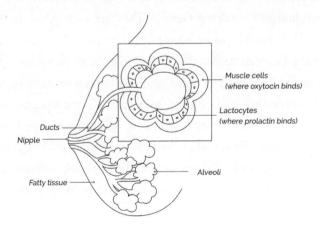

Muscle cells
(where oxytocin binds)

Lactocytes
(where prolactin binds)

Ducts

Nipple

Alveoli

Fatty tissue

Women's breasts are made of two kinds of tissue: fatty tissue and breast tissue. The breast tissue is the part that changes during pregnancy in response to the hormone estrogen so it can make milk. When a woman is not pregnant, the amount of fatty tissue in her breasts can make them look large, even if they don't have a lot of breast tissue. During pregnancy, a woman's breasts change from having more fatty tissue to having more specialized breast tissue, usually by twenty-two weeks. The size of a woman's breasts alone doesn't tell you how much of each tissue they contain. Accordingly, you can't tell how much milk a woman's breasts are able to make just by looking at them.

Most breast tissue sits right under your areola, where your baby latches on, and is made up of two types of structures: *alveoli,* the round structures where milk is made and stored, and *ducts,* the little tubes where milk travels from the alveoli to the nipple and out the breast. During pregnancy, the alveoli have two layers. The inner lining changes into cells that make milk, called *lactocytes.* The outer layers become tiny muscle cells that can *squeeze* milk out of the alveoli.[5] Think of each alveoli as an individual milk-making factory. They are each generally the same size, but the more alveoli a breast has, the more milk-making factories it has, and the more milk it can make. Each breast can have more or less alveoli, which is why some breasts make more milk than others, even in the same woman. And these alveoli develop in response to the hormone prolactin, which we will discuss when we talk about your milk supply.

Often not talked about are the little glands around your nipples, called *Montgomery glands.* During pregnancy they swell and start making a waxy substance that doesn't even have a name, which is surprising given how important it is. That waxy substance is how your baby "finds" your breast when he's first born and until his other senses catch up to his sense of smell (see Chapter 4).

How Lactating Breasts Release Milk

When your baby is nursing, your breasts are helping too. But the only way they can is if your baby is latched on correctly and it feels good to you. That pleasant sensation of him nursing is important, because it stimulates little receptors on your nipple and areola, which in turn make your brain release hormones. The main hormone your brain releases in response to pleasant nursing is oxytocin, or the feel-good hormone. It's the same hormone people release when they fall in love.

Oxytocin is a wonderful hormone that does a bunch of things in a new mom.[6] It helps your uterus shrink down to pre-pregnancy size. It gives you a sense of calm and bliss, literally making you fall in love with your baby (known as *physiologic bonding*). It also travels back to your breast to stimulate those tiny muscle cells around the alveoli to squeeze out the milk. This "squeezing out" is called the milk ejection reflex, or let-down.[7] An interesting thing about those little muscle cells is that they will contract *only* when oxytocin stimulates them. Nothing else makes them squeeze out milk. Given that oxytocin is released only from pleasant emotional or physical sensations, then it follows that . . .

good feeling on your breasts = release of oxytocin = good letdown

bad/painful feeling on your breasts =
no release of oxytocin = no letdown

Your letdown starts thirty to forty-five seconds after your baby latches on, because it takes time for your hormones to get circulating. The letdown can last anywhere from forty-five seconds to three and a half minutes, and happens more than once in a nursing session. For some women it can happen four times! After the first letdown, more than half of the milk in your breast is pushed out. After the second, half of what is left is released. If you consider the timing, if you have an average supply, you should be able to empty each breast after about ten to fifteen minutes. If you nurse longer than that, your baby may not be getting much milk and is probably soothing or passing out.[8] Prolonged nursing may also mean that something is wrong, especially if it is painful (more on this in Chapter 6).

Without a letdown, it's hard to get milk out of your breasts, because a lot of milk stays trapped in your alveoli. That's why pumping doesn't empty every woman's breasts out the way an effectively nursing baby can. It is also why pain, which prevents oxytocin release, also prevents your breasts from pushing out the milk. In other words, *nursing through pain makes your breasts hold on to milk.* Even moms with full breasts can't empty them when they experience pain. Some moms' breasts are so dependent on oxytocin that they won't release milk no matter how full they are. It may seem confusing if your breasts are leaking all over the place. But if you have a lot of milk and it stays trapped in your breasts, your breasts will stop making it.

You could also end up with plugged ducts and breast infections (more on this in Chapters 9 and 10).

Patient Perspective

Sara was a second-time mother with a two-week-old baby.

"I have very little milk," she said, with a look of responsibility and pain. "It was the same with my first child. It's my fault, but the lactation consultant told me to come anyway just to check."

Sara wanted to nurse more than anything and was prepared to suffer for it. And suffer she did. She nursed right away in the hospital, every two hours, as she was told, to "maximize" her supply. Although it hurt, and her nipples bled, she persevered. She was determined to do everything she could to breastfeed this baby after failing with her first. But already two weeks in, her baby wasn't gaining weight, and his bilirubin was creeping up.

"The pediatrician told me to give him formula. But I wanted to see you first. I know I have some milk, but he wants to nurse all the time. I pump a little afterward, so I know he's getting some." Fear crept into her voice. Fear that she was starving her baby and shame that she was being selfish in wanting to nurse. She didn't want to give her baby formula, because formula meant giving up.

What Sara didn't know is that nursing through pain sends a reverse signal to the brain of nursing mothers. The common advice of continuing to nurse even though it hurts so the baby doesn't "forget" the breast goes against physiology. It simultaneously makes the mother's brain secrete a hormone that prevents milk ejection and teaches the baby that the breast is a difficult food source. In following well-meant advice, Sara was actually *creating* a low-supply situation for herself.

How Your Milk Supply Is Established and Maintained

Your milk supply has to first be established, and then it has to be maintained. The way this happens is complicated and timely. There are a lot of variables that change every day for the first four weeks of breastfeeding, so every day counts. Here, assume I am describing a full-term baby and a mom who is an average milk producer without any medical problems. Keep in mind, breastfeeding experiences greatly differ depending on your actual supply, which we will discuss in Chapter 11.

During the first few days after your baby is born, your breasts make colostrum. This is the nutrient-rich "pre-milk" that is produced in small amounts (20 to 40 mL a day). Because your baby has been waterlogged from being in your womb for so long, colostrum is all he needs at first. On Days 3 to 4, your breasts start making *transitional milk,* which is exactly what it sounds like. It is the milk that changes every day until it eventually becomes *mature breastmilk.* On Days 3 to 4, your breasts produce 300 to 400 milliliters a day, and that rapidly increases by Day 5 to around 500 to 800 milliliters a day of transitional milk. By Days 10 to 14 your breasts are making mature breastmilk. The total amount of milk a mom can produce is widely variable, and by widely, I mean anywhere from 800 milliliters to thousands of milliliters a day. In general, your breasts will produce 800 to 1,000 milliliters a day, which is enough to feed your baby from four weeks onward.

Your milk supply starts out small and rapidly increases over the first two to three weeks. By four weeks, your breasts will make the same amount of milk per day that they will be making at six months. In other words, by the time your baby is four weeks old, the *total volume* of milk he needs remains the same, even as he is growing. He may nurse less often when he is bigger, but he will also take in more milk with each session.

The Foundation of Your Milk Supply

Setting up your milk supply is most important in the first two to three weeks. The hormone prolactin plays a huge role in this.[9] Prolactin makes your breast tissue turn into milk-making factories (alveoli). More alveoli means your breasts will be able to produce more milk at any given time. Prolactin is released by the pituitary gland in your brain and increases ten-to-twenty-fold during pregnancy. After your baby is born, as long as you nurse, the levels stay high for the first few weeks, but they also fluctuate throughout the day. But nursing has to feel good for prolactin to be released. In other words, pleasant sensations on your nipples mean more prolactin for your breasts.

After the first few weeks of nursing, your prolactin levels go back down to pre-pregnancy levels. This means your breasts have the greatest chance of forming milk-making factories—and developing the ability to make more milk—in the first few weeks. After that, it is much harder to increase your total milk supply.

Prolactin has another role. It creates more receptors on the alveoli. Think of receptors as "on" buttons. When prolactin binds to its receptors, it tells the alveoli to make more milk for the next nursing session. The more prolactin you have in your bloodstream in the first few weeks, the more alveoli you'll have, and more receptors will be on those alveoli. With all those alveoli, your breasts can more easily be "turned on" to make milk. This is important, because after a few weeks, your brain will stop making as much prolactin, even if you are breastfeeding. So the window of making more alveoli closes after the first three to four weeks. But if you already have a lot of alveoli, you only need a little prolactin to stimulate your breasts to make a lot of milk.

Timing is so important. Because of the way prolactin works, nursing normally for the first few weeks allows your breasts to make more milk for the whole duration of nursing. It's important to identify problems early on if you want to protect your supply. If your baby isn't nursing well or if you nurse through pain during the first few weeks, your window of greatest milk production can be missed.[10] This situation is unfair and frustrating, because the first few weeks of breastfeeding are also the most confusing and overwhelming. Things change on a daily basis, but you can't waste time with inaccurate information. If you take the "wait and see" approach, you may not be able to make up for what you've lost. When it comes to breastfeeding, most things are time dependent.

Maintenance of Your Milk Supply

After the first few weeks, your breasts will have the same number of milk-making factories they are going to have for the whole time you are nursing. This means your *milk-making capacity* (the maximum amount of milk your breasts can hold at any given time) is set by about four weeks. But the total amount of milk your breasts can *produce* in a day depends on three things:

1. How often you empty your breasts
2. How quickly you empty your breasts
3. How completely you empty your breasts

Let's talk about supply and demand. Your milk supply is regulated both by the amount of milk that is emptied from your breasts and by the amount of milk left behind. Remember, your alveoli are milk-making factories. They have receptors that bind to prolactin, which are "on" buttons that cause them to make more milk. When the alveoli are full of milk, those receptors are stretched out and deformed so prolactin can't "turn them on." When your alveoli are empty, prolactin can connect easily to the receptors, so your alveoli can make more milk. The net result is that empty breasts make more milk than full ones.

Your breasts have another way of controlling how much milk you make with a protein called *feedback inhibitor of lactation,* or *FIL*.[11] FIL is made by alveoli when they make milk, so the more milk your breasts make, the more FIL there is in your milk. In other words, fuller breasts not only have more milk, but also have more FIL. When the amount of FIL builds up, it prevents your alveoli from making more milk and breaks down prolactin receptors. So the longer the breast remains full of milk, the longer it is also full of FIL, and the less milk it will make. When your milk gets emptied from your breasts, so does FIL.

FIL is important so your breasts can limit how full they can get. If you didn't have FIL, your breasts could get over-full and your alveoli could break down. FIL also fine-tunes and controls the amount of milk each breast can make. FIL is why the same mom sometimes makes different amounts of milk in each breast. It is also why removing a slow stream of a small amount of milk will, over time, reduce your overall supply.

The bottom line? Full breasts make less milk than empty ones. Not only that, but the more quickly you empty them (e.g., ten minutes instead of an hour) and the more often you empty them out, the more they will fill up again.

The Nutritional Components of Breastmilk

Your milk is customized. It changes based on foods you eat and the time of day. Where you live and the kinds of bacteria and viruses you are exposed to also have an effect. But even if you don't have perfect nutrition or take supplements, your body will do its best to give your baby what he needs.

A quick note about *foremilk* and *hindmilk*. Breasts make only one kind of milk. It has a thick, fatty component and a more watery, sugary component. The fatty component often sludges behind, getting stuck in the alveoli and ducts because it's so dense. The sugary component is more lightweight, so it floats upstream to the ducts and nipples. When a baby latches, he gets the sugary *foremilk* first, followed by the fatty *hindmilk* when the letdown happens. If you pump out your milk and let it sit in a bottle, the fatty part of the milk floats to the top. Also, breastmilk can have different "hues," like yellow, bluish, or greenish. I've even seen orange breastmilk. Even though it looks weird, all this is normal.

Regardless of what you eat, breastmilk is generally made up of the following:

Calories—60–75 kcal/100 mL
Water—90 g/100 mL water, or 87%
Protein—0.8–1.3 g/100 mL of protein, 30% casein
    and 70% whey, or 7%

Whey proteins are liquid and include alpha lactalbumin, lactoferrin, lysozyme, serum albumin, secretory immunoglobulin IgA (sIgA), insulin, epidermal growth factor (EGF), and many enzymes. Most of these proteins are found only in human milk, not animal milk. These proteins do things like help with your baby's immune system, provide nutrition, and make other proteins active. Some help protect your baby's gut from infections, whether they are bacterial, viral, or fungal.

Casein is the more solid protein and is less digestible than whey. Human breastmilk has a lot less casein than most animal milks. For example, cow's milk has 82 percent casein and 18 percent whey. Too much casein can overwhelm your baby's maturing kidneys. Cow's milk also has a protein called beta-lactoglobulin that babies can't digest. This is why babies often get colic and tummy upset from cow's-milk-based formulas. Some babies are allergic to all milk proteins.

Sugar—6.9 to 7.4 g/100 mL, of which 90 to 95% is
    lactose, or 1%

Lactose is a sugar, and it is mostly used as calories. But some isn't digested and makes a baby's stool softer. There is one type of sugar, oligosaccharide, that controls the kind of bacterial strains that grow in your baby's gut and help protect against infections. This sugar is important because it feeds the healthy bacteria in your baby's gut, called the microbiome. This sugary part of breastmilk (the foremilk) is made in your alveoli, but it floats up to the ducts, because it isn't as heavy as the hindmilk.

Fat—3 to 5 g/100 mL, mostly in the form of palmitic
    and oleic acids, or 4%

Fats provide half the calories in your milk. The fat content in your milk varies throughout the day and increases over time the longer you breastfeed. Although all the components of milk are made in the alveoli, fats are heavier and tend to stick behind, so your baby has to get through the sugary parts before getting to the fats. This fatty hindmilk sludges behind. When your baby gets the hindmilk, the fat in his small intestine tell his brain to release a hormone that makes him stop eating and fall asleep (see Chapter 4). Certain fatty acids—DHA (docosahexaeonic acid) and ARA (arachidonic acid)—are found only in breastmilk, not animal milk, and they are very important in your baby's brain and eye development.

Vitamins and Minerals—0.2 g/100mL in total

Your breastmilk has the following vitamins and minerals:

- 200 mg /100 mL sodium
- 25 mg/100 mL calcium
- 9 mg/100 mL phosphorus
- 5 mg/100 mL vitamin C
- 3.5 mg/100 mL magnesium
- Smaller amounts of iron, copper, zinc, vitamin A, pantothenic acid, nicotinic acid, iodine, and vitamins K, D, E, and B

Your milk has very little iron and a small amount of zinc that decreases over time. Thankfully, your baby is born with enough iron to last for the first six months. He should get the extra zinc and iron he needs through food when he starts eating solids at six months. The same isn't true of vitamin D. We mostly get vitamin D via the sun, and your milk runs out of it, so your pediatrician will recommend you give your baby extra vitamin D when he turns six months.

Cellular Elements

Breastmilk contains lots of living cells. Most of them are active immune cells that are customized by your breasts based on your baby's saliva. Others are stem cells that help your baby in the future. You also pass on genetic information through your milk that turns genes on and off in your baby.

Now that you understand the mechanics of the separate elements (baby and breast), let's talk about how they interact.

Dulce de Latché:
Baby Meets Breast

Although it may seem simple on the surface, breastfeeding is more than just putting your nipple in your baby's mouth and letting her suck. It is as beautiful as it is complex, and when it works properly, it's easy to see why everyone is such a fan.

When we hear the word *breastfeeding,* we think of the *act* of breastfeeding. But what we don't think about is everything that has to come together to make it happen. First off, there are two people involved: you and your baby. Although each of you has a doctor who is looking out for you individually, there isn't a medical specialty for both of you together. You have your obstetrician, and your baby has her pediatrician. When you go to the doctor, they will most like consider you and your baby separately. But breastfeeding is all about the "unit."

In this chapter we will take what we learned from Chapter 3 and put it into context, breaking down the important parts so you can really understand how the whole process works. When this "machine" is working perfectly, it is incredibly cool.

The Mechanics of Breastfeeding

FINDING THE BREAST

When babies are first born, they are functionally blind. They sense the world through touch and mostly smell. The smell they are most strongly programmed to find is also their most likely source of food: your breasts. The Montgomery glands in your nipples produce a waxy substance that has a particular smell.[1] The smell is very potent for your baby, and guides her to your breasts. Babies are known to crawl up their mom's breasts to find it. The smell also triggers your baby to open her mouth wide and gape when she gets there.

THE GAPE

We discussed the gape a little in Chapter 3, but I'd like to go into a little more detail here. The gape is the most important part of breastfeeding, because without it, breastfeeding can't happen normally. Gaping is an actual unhinging of your baby's jaw so she can open her mouth very wide and keep it open without having to hold it open. The gape is a relaxed position, so your baby doesn't waste precious energy trying to open wide instead of working to pull milk out of your breasts. It is not simply hinging at the jaw, which takes effort.

The gape is a reflex, which means it is automatic. Your baby will gape if you bring her chin to the skin near your breast. She will also gape if you touch her chin, or she smells your breast. It happens very fast, so it is hard to measure. It may seem like your baby is gaping, but you won't know for sure until you latch her on to your breast and it *feels* right. When she is gaped, she should be able to fit all your nipple and most of your areola into her mouth.

If your baby tries to latch on and can't get any milk out of your breast repeatedly, she will eventually lose her gape reflex. Also, because the gape is automatic, if she doesn't gape normally, it means she *can't* gape normally. It is also important to know the difference between the gape reflex and the *rooting reflex*. The rooting reflex is when your baby turns her head to the side and opens her mouth a little when you touch her cheek. She usually does this more often when she's hungry.

THE PERFECT LATCH

Before you latch your baby on, you should "prime" your breast to get the milk flowing and get your nipple ready. One great way to do it is described by Dr. Jane Morton on the Stanford Medical School website.[2] Place your forefinger and thumb directly across from each other on your areola. Then press them down, toward your chest, and pull them together to meet just outside your nipple. Do it several times until the milk that's sitting in your surface ducts comes out of your nipple. Now you are ready for your baby.

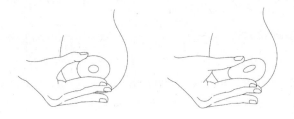

I'm going to describe what I've seen to be the best way to latch your baby on. Obviously, there are many ways to breastfeed. There are even entire books on all the different positions and latches. Think of this one as a fail-safe latch. It is the simplest, most effective way to make sure your baby is latched on correctly and able to pull milk out of your breast. If you and your baby can master this latch, you can use any latch and any position you want and it will work. If you can't master it, that's a red flag that something is wrong. Without a good latch, none of the "rules" of breastfeeding apply.

Use the below images for reference as I describe the steps.

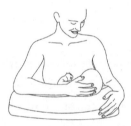

Figure 1: Lay baby across pillow

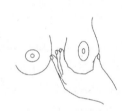

Figure 2: Cup breast with a U hold

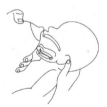

Figure 3: Hold baby, nose to breast

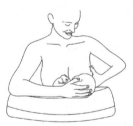

Figure 4: Latch on baby to breast, maintain cross-cradle hold

Sit on a chair, preferably with side arms, or a couch. Make sure you have good back support, because you are not going to lean forward to breastfeed. Place a regular pillow on your lap and your Boppy pillow on top of that. If you are using a My Brest Friend pillow, it should be high enough. You can even use a combination of pillows, like a Boppy and Little Beam or a Butterfly pillow. Lay your baby across the pillow with her head next to the breast you want to nurse from. Now you are ready to start.

First, form your hand into a U. It should be the hand on the same side as your breast. Cup your breast from underneath and squeeze your thumb and fingers together, flattening your breast. Make sure to grab your breast as far away from your areola as possible, even resting your hand against your chest wall. You want as much free areola as possible to get as much as you can into your baby's mouth. Hold your breast that way, keeping your nipple pointing up, not down.

Next, hold your baby's head with your opposite hand by putting your forefinger and thumb behind her ears, around the base of her head and neck. Bring your baby's *nose* to your nipple so she can smell it. The smell of your breast will make her open her mouth and gape. Once she gapes, quickly align her lower lip to the edge of your areola and push her wide-open mouth over your nipple and down onto your breast. It will happen fast, so you may have to try a few times before you get it. Even though you may be tempted, don't lean down and put your breast into her mouth. Not only will this hurt your back, but it will also make it harder to get her whole mouth around your areola.

Once she is on your breast, her mouth should fit over your whole nipple and most of your areola. Your nipple should be all the way in the back of her throat so you can't feel anything touching it. The farthest edge of your areola should be sitting between her upper gum and her tongue. From the outside, her upper and lower lip should be flanged out, but it's easier to see the upper lip. As long as it feels good, you don't have to actually look at the lower lip. Now your baby is latched on.

SUCK AND SWALLOW

Once your baby is latched correctly, the roof of her mouth, her hard palate, will be filled with your breast. As we learned in Chapter 2, this will trigger her *suck reflex.* She will lift the front part of her tongue up and compress your breast against the roof of her mouth. Then she will pull her tongue to the back of her throat. This compression and pulling of her tongue moves the milk forward through your milk ducts and prevents backflow. It also stretches your nipple and areola to one and half times their original size, so over time, breastfeeding actually changes the shape of your nipples. If breastfeeding feels good, your nipples will eventually custom-fit your baby's mouth. If it hurts, it means she isn't latched on deeply, so she will compress and pinch your nipple into a lipstick shape (see Chapter 10).

Now, with her tongue in the back of her throat, her *swallow reflex* takes over. Her jaw will drop to create a vacuum, pulling more milk out of your breasts. The milk will pour out your nipple and into her esophagus, and she will swallow. For added protection, her soft palate will lift up and close off her nasal cavity so milk doesn't come out of her nose. Her voice box, or larynx, will also move up and forward to prevent milk from going into her trachea and lungs.

And the whole suck-swallow cycle will begin again.

Remember that your baby's suck reflex will kick in no matter what presses against the roof of her mouth. Your finger, a pacifier, a bottle—anything that stimulates the roof of her mouth will make her suck. Conversely, if the roof of her mouth is high, or your breast can't get all the way inside her mouth, she may not suck at all.

THE LETDOWN

After 30 to 45 seconds of feel-good sucking and swallowing, your brain will release the hormone oxytocin. Oxytocin travels through your bloodstream to your breasts and makes those little muscle cells around the milk-making factories squeeze out more milk, triggering the letdown. To conserve the milk in your other breast, it happens only on the breast your baby is nursing on. Your other breast may leak, but it won't pour out like the nursing side, so your breast can save that milk for when your baby is ready.

The letdown sometimes doesn't happen when you pump, because oxytocin is mostly released from your brain when you have a pleasant sensation on your areola. This "positive pressure" that happens from your baby compressing and pulling her tongue across your areola combined with your oxytocin pushing out the milk is the main way your breasts empty. The "negative pressure" of the vacuum created when your baby drops her jaw is only a small part of milk removal. Pumps use only negative pressure, or a vacuum, to pull milk out of your breast. It's no wonder they don't work the same for every mom and some moms can't get any milk out by using a pump alone.

HOLDING YOUR BREAST IN POSITION

Once your baby is nursing, you need to make sure your breast stays where it is. When you and your baby "fit" well, the only friction you should feel is your baby's tongue on your breast and areola. You shouldn't feel anything on your nipple. Your nipple should sit all the way in the back of her throat and not move at all. No moving means no friction. No friction means no pain. The more of your breast that fills your baby's mouth, the easier it is to maintain that deep latch. Depending on your breast shape and size and your baby's "fit," you may be able to let go of your breast and just let your baby nurse.

Sometimes, to keep everything stable, you will need to hold your breast with one hand and your baby's head with the other. You can even prop her head up with a rolled-up burping cloth or blanket. Some newborns won't have enough strength to hold a heavy breast in their mouths at first. This could be because of their mom's breast shape, weight, size, fullness, and so on. For example, if you have a large, heavy breast, even if your baby is latched on deeply, your breast may slide out of her mouth from sheer weight alone. Similarly, if you have flatter breasts that are firm because they are full of milk, your baby may not be able to get enough of a "bite." You won't have to do it forever. Over time, your baby's mouth muscles, also called *sucking pads,* will get strong enough that she can hold your breast in her mouth without help. (Interesting fact: Babies who breastfeed have stronger sucking pads than those who only bottle-feed.) But if you latch your baby on and she keeps slipping off your breast, try holding your breast first before jumping to interventions. Remember: The goal is to minimize friction and stabilize the whole system.

POSTURE AND HOW THE LATCH SHOULD LOOK

When your baby is latched on, you should be able to lean back to support your back and pull the pillows toward you to support your baby. You shouldn't lean forward. Also, be aware of how much tension you are holding in the rest of your body. If your shoulders are raised, relax them. If you are squeezing your breast too tightly, relax your fingers. If your toes are curling from pain, then something is wrong. Stop immediately and try to relatch your baby. If you try to relatch and it hurts no matter what you do, it's better to stop the session, pump, try a bottle, and ask for help. Don't push through the pain.

When you look down from above, your baby should look peaceful but be actively sucking. You'll probably be able to see only her side profile, which means she is in the right position. She should be able to breathe out the sides of her nostrils, even though her nose is pushed against your breast. If you watch carefully, you can see her swallowing. The soft part of her throat, beneath her chin, should expand for a split second each time the milk goes down her esophagus. Her neck should be at a 90-degree angle to her jaw, not bent forward. This angle gives her enough room to pull her jaw down and create an internal vacuum when she swallows. If her neck is too extended or stretched out, she won't be able to use her neck muscles to help her swallow. Sometimes she will suck a few times then swallow, and sometimes she will swallow every time she sucks.

It can be deceptive if she is sucking and sucking but only swallowing a few times. She shouldn't be working that hard. Similarly, if she sucks a little, then falls asleep, try to wake her up to keep her active on the breast. Sometimes premature babies fall asleep because their reflexes aren't fully active yet. Jaundice, which is common in newborns, can also make your baby sleepy. Even though babies take breaks during nursing sessions, if your baby is latched on but not actively nursing, it doesn't count as breastfeeding.

How Long Should Breastfeeding Take?

With a perfect latch, nursing should take ten to fifteen minutes on each breast and your baby should want to eat every two to three hours. These are average times that can fluctuate from day to day and throughout the day. As your baby gets older, the time it takes to nurse should get shorter, and the time between nursing sessions should get longer. That's because your supply increases during the first month and your baby should get better at getting your milk.

Many in the breastfeeding community may disagree because they don't like committing to numbers and timing. But hear me out. Every mom-and-baby dyad is different. Some babies eat for longer or shorter times because every mom has a different milk supply and letdown. But numbers give us a frame of reference. Without a frame of reference, it's easy to group everything together on the spectrum of normal instead of identifying that something is wrong.

For example, if your baby nurses for twenty minutes instead of fifteen, fine. If she goes two hours instead of three hours, fine. But if she latches on for an hour and gets hungry an hour after you nurse, something is wrong. It shouldn't take her that long, and if it does, not only is she working too hard, but she also isn't emptying your breasts fast enough for them to fill up again for the next feed. If it goes on for days or weeks, you could lose your milk supply and your baby could lose weight.

Conversely, if you have a huge supply, your baby may only nurse for five minutes every two hours. While she may still gain a lot of weight, she may only be getting the sugary foremilk, not the fatty hindmilk, so she never feels full. It may also give her watery stools and make her gassy and spit up a lot.

If timing and numbers aren't your thing and you want to make sure your baby is getting enough to eat, take a step back and look at the big picture. As long as she is gaining weight and has the right number of wet and soiled diapers a day (see page 202), and you are pain-free with breasts that fill up before nursing and are empty after nursing, you're on the right track.

Do You Always Have to Breastfeed?

There is a myth that if you breastfeed, you should always offer your breast before a bottle so your baby doesn't "forget" it. This will not happen. It's also not true that if you give your baby a bottle, she will choose the bottle over you. So why have these beliefs been propagated for so long? I chalk it up to a misunderstanding of cause and effect.

First of all, your baby can't forget your breast. She is hardwired to find it through her reflexes. Skin-to-skin contact makes both of you release oxytocin and bond to each other. The sound of your voice makes her want to search for you (even if she can't see at first). The way you smell, especially that waxy substance around your nipples, helps her "find" your breasts. These reflexes are important, because babies want to survive, and to survive they need food and protection—both of which come from you. The best way to mess it up is by teaching your baby to ignore her reflexes. This happens more often than you think, although usually with the best of intentions.

Avoiding early skin-to-skin contact is one way. Unlike in the past, when doctors purposefully separated moms and babies, nowadays this only happens for medical reasons. C-sections can delay skin-to-skin. Fetal distress or your baby needing immediate medical care is another cause. Prematurity and/or the need for NICU treatment limits or even prevents your physical contact with her.

Another way to teach your baby to stop choosing your breast is to override her reflexes. Silicone nipples and plastic bottles don't mean anything to your baby unless she *learns* to choose them over you. How does this happen? One way is to breastfeed her repeatedly when she isn't getting milk from you (your supply may not have come in or she can't transfer milk), then follow it up with a bottle of formula or breastmilk. When she smells your breast, nurses, and doesn't get food, she will *learn* that your breast won't feed her. When you follow that up with a bottle because she needs to eat, she will learn that the bottle means food. Repeat this over and over again, and before you know it, she will *learn* that the smell of your breast means no food but the feel of the silicone nipple means lots of food. Very quickly, she will start to choose the bottle over you. (This is also called nipple aversion, which we will discuss in Chapter 12.)

The bottom line is that if your baby is able to nurse normally and get milk from you, it will feel good for both of you. If you give her a bottle once in a while, she won't automatically choose the bottle over you. In fact, a lot of babies reject bottles given by their mom because they want milk directly from the source. Even if your baby learns to avoid your breasts, you can usually retrain her to come back.

The Experience of Breastfeeding

There are three basic parts in breastfeeding:

1. Your baby must be able to get the milk out of your breast (the act of breastfeeding).

2. You have to have a good milk supply.

3. Your baby must want to go to your breast.

Although each part may seem simple on its own, all three are intricately connected and dependent on one another. For example, if your baby can't easily pull milk out of your breast, your supply will drop unless you pump. If you have a low supply, your baby will eventually get frustrated or quit nursing. You may have plenty of milk, but if she can't pull it out, she'll cry when she gets near it. We tend to focus on the smaller parts of breastfeeding. But you have to stand back and take a look at the bigger picture.

A pleasant latch with normal suck, swallow, and letdown results in the most efficient milk transfer out of your breast and into your baby. This series of events informs every other outcome in breastfeeding. If your baby can't latch on correctly and pull out the milk, and your breasts don't push out the milk, then none of the "rules" of breastfeeding apply.

But don't worry just yet. We're going to go step by step through the first and most important months of breastfeeding so you have a complete understanding of the process.

PART TWO

The Milky Way: A Week-by-Week Guide to the First Three Months of Breastfeeding

Congrats! You Just Had A Baby. Now What?

You've just had a baby. Now you will need to figure out how to feed him, and you will need to do so in the dizzying time after you give birth, when you likely just want to take a nap. Whether you're parsing the advice from your rushed meeting with a busy lactation consultant in the hospital or struggling to figure out how read all your baby's cues after a home birth, this chapter will answer everything you need to know as you start nursing. We will talk about how the type of delivery affects nursing, and what kind of support is available to you. We will also talk about how to deal with the rapid succession of advice from doctors, lactation consultants, and nurses on the maternity ward, and the differences between hospital and home birth. But first, allow me to share . . .

My Story

The morning my daughter was born, the nurse wheeled her into my hospital room, all bundled up in a blanket. My first thought was "She's so beautiful." My second thought was "Why are they trusting me with this tiny, helpless human?" I had spent so much time preparing for the delivery, I hadn't pictured our first moments alone together. I had no idea what to do.

She was born around two o'clock in the morning, so I had had very little sleep. The delivery wasn't quite what I'd expected. I had planned for a vaginal birth with no drugs—that part I got. What I hadn't anticipated was my rapid transition from closed cervix to full dilation in less than an hour. I also hadn't prepared for the fact that her cord would be wrapped around her neck so that every time I pushed, her heart rate dropped. When it was time to get her out of me, I was relieved when the on-call obstetrician wheeled in a cart of medical equipment. In my delirium, I had assumed I was finally getting the epidural I had originally refused. I was wrong about that too. Instead, the obstetrician held up a huge metallic spatula-looking thing. Then he uttered the most honest words any doctor has ever said to me: "This is going to hurt worse than anything you've ever felt before." Pain like the color red filled my brain, and, with one sustained push, my baby was out. She was healthy, and, despite the shock, so was I.

A nurse brought her to meet me, laying her on my chest for a few moments before whisking her away for a bath. It was brief, but sweet. I passed out while I was getting stitched up, thankful for the few drops of Demerol I was finally given for pain.

That was the last thing I remember before waking up in my

hospital room. I was a whole new person. I was a mom. And my baby, capped and swaddled, was perfect. And that perfect angel was crying and sticking her hands in her mouth. Sleep deprived, a little drugged, and emotionally raw, I wondered what she needed. Then, right on cue, my breasts started leaking. I was a mom. And being a mom meant breastfeeding my baby.

Breastfeeding had always been my plan. My mom nursed me for more than two years. When I was growing up, she used to brag about her nonstop supply, and how she fattened up each of her four babies to epic proportions. Even though nursing was out of vogue at the time, she was adamant about doing it because, for her, breastfeeding was synonymous with motherhood. My sisters and numerous friends had similar perspectives and experiences. It had never crossed my mind that my journey would be any different.

I picked up my baby to calm her, then sat on the bed. Assuming breastfeeding was as obvious as I'd been told, I pulled out my breast and held her to it. After a few minutes she opened her mouth and latched on. It hurt. Not as much as the birth, but close. Milk was coming out the sides of her mouth, so I assumed everything was fine. After a few minutes, she stopped sucking, but I kept her on my breast. The little I had read about breastfeeding mentioned that it was important to have lots of skin-to-skin contact, so I kept her latched on. The pain was a surprise, but I figured it was just like the birth: No pain, no gain.

A labor and delivery nurse popped her head in to check on us. "Looks like you're doing great," she said.

"Is it supposed to hurt?" I asked, worried I was being whiny.

"No, it's supposed to feel good, but it also hurts. It's part of the whole toughening-up process," she assured me.

I didn't like the thought of my nipples "toughening up," but what did I know? As the day went on, my breasts seemed fuller and my baby kept nursing. Even though my nipples got more and more sore, my daughter didn't seem to mind. In fact, she was clearly in love with them, because every time I tried to take her off, she cried. By the next morning, I got so used to the gnawing pain in my breasts I started to believe it was a sign of love.

In wasn't until day two, when my nipples started bleeding, that I questioned the whole breastfeeding thing. Desperate for a nap, I let the nurses give her a bottle. After her feed, she slept for three whole hours. I was shocked. She never slept that long after I fed her. I was happy for her but jealous for me. I didn't want her to love the bottle more than my breasts, so I became even more determined in my efforts. Despite the pain and long feeding sessions, I breastfed her continuously until we were discharged home.

In the hospital, every nurse told me how great we were doing. Even the pediatrician was pleased with our progress. I felt like a superhero, and I had the destroyed nipples to prove it.

It wasn't until we visited the pediatrician the following week that I had cause for alarm. My daughter had lost more weight than she should have. Without asking about my supply or feeding schedule, she told me I had to start supplementing with formula. I had no choice but to comply.

Your Birth Story

This kind of blurry haze is pretty common when you give birth. The one thing all births have in common is that no matter how much you plan, you can never be sure how yours will end up. It can start one way and end up another. Home births may turn into hospital births, and vaginal births may turn into C-sections. The best birth is one where both mom and baby are healthy. If you get the birth you wanted, wonderful! But even if you don't, you can adapt to your circumstances and still start off on the right foot when it comes to breastfeeding.

Start thinking about the possible birth outcomes when you are still pregnant. Don't make assumptions. Ask a lot of questions but remember: Not all advice is created equal. If something doesn't resonate with you, don't take it as a hard truth. And most of all, trust your intuition.

IN THE WOMB WHERE IT HAPPENS

Womb position is something that is rarely talked about when it comes to breastfeeding. Surprisingly, it can have the greatest impact. The way your baby sits in your womb determines the shape of his body, and the biggest part of his body is his head. Most of the time, babies move around during your whole pregnancy until the last few weeks, when they go head down and stay there until the delivery. When babies move around a lot, their head shape is rounder and their jaws are only set back a little. But sometimes your baby ends up in one position early and stays there for most of the third trimester. This time is also when he is growing the most and the fastest, so his head shape becomes molded by the rigid structures around it, namely your ribs and pelvis.[1]

For example, if your baby stays on his side at the end of the third trimester, he is in what is called the *breech position.* His head is tucked up under your rib cage, so as it grows, it will be shaped accordingly.[2] Similarly, if he goes head down *early* in your third trimester, his head will be shaped like the inside of your pelvic girdle. Because of the way your pelvis is shaped, his head will be more oblong. The axis of his head will be more vertical than round, which affects the way all his head and neck structures are able to move. Depending on how deep down he sits in your pelvis, this position may make your delivery easier, but it usually makes breastfeeding harder.

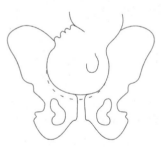

Figure 1: Head down, not engaged, rounder head shape

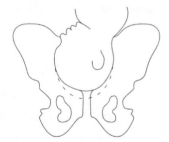

Figure 2: Head down, engaged, oblong head shape

Doctors of osteopathy (DOs) and cranial osteopathy are very familiar with how womb position affects head shape, and they talk about it in their teachings. However, medical doctors (MDs) think about head shape a different way. They describe it as based on the way your baby is born.[3] For example, if your baby is born vaginally, his tiny skull bones have to overlap so he can fit through your birth canal. If a vacuum or forceps is used for delivery, he can get bruises, and his skull bones may also shift. In both cases, his skull bones will "right" themselves in the days to weeks after he is born, but the same isn't true of how his head forms in the womb. That shape is more permanent.

Your baby's head shape is one of the most important predictors of how hard or easy it will be to nurse him. If you understand how your baby's head shape *in the womb* affects his ability to breastfeed, you can even be prepared before you give birth (see Chapter 10).

DELIVERY TYPE

The way your baby is born can also affect your initial breastfeeding experience. I will go over the basics, but you should also speak to your obstetrician about delivery options and how delivery methods can promote breastfeeding or make it more challenging.

Spontaneous vaginal births are the most common and the simplest. This is when you give birth without drugs that make you go into labor, and no vacuum or forceps are used to help your baby come out. These kinds of births can happen anywhere—at home, in the hospital, in a car on the way to the hospital, etc. Water deliveries also fall under this category. Many women work with midwives and doulas to help them through this often long and painful process. You have the option of getting an epidural for pain or going drug-free. For some women, however, these kinds of births are not possible. You should discuss your options with your obstetrician.

In terms of breastfeeding, spontaneous births are the gold standard. If your baby is also full term, your hormones will be in sync with your delivery so your breasts will already be making milk. Your baby's reflexes will be active. When your baby travels through your birth canal, he will get coated with the bacteria that will form his gut microbiome. That microbiome will be fed best by your breastmilk. You and your baby will have immediate skin-to-skin contact, which gets oxytocin flowing in both of you. Some women even nurse right away, as soon as their baby comes out.

Induced vaginal births are a little different. These births happen the same way as regular vaginal births, but you are given medicine to make it happen sooner and/or faster. There is usually a safety reason for this, like your labor isn't progressing after your water breaks, or your baby is overdue. If you have this kind of birth, depending on how far you are into the pregnancy, it can make breastfeeding a little more challenging. If your baby comes early, your hormones may not be synced up to the birth, so your milk supply may be delayed. Similarly, your baby's reflexes may not be awake enough yet, so he may be sleepy when it comes to feeding.

You can have a vaginal birth after a previous C-section, but, depending on your circumstances, that birth will fall under one of the two mentioned above.

Even though breastfeeding after a vaginal birth gives you some advantages, it isn't perfect. Sometimes labor takes a long time and you can simply be too exhausted to nurse. Or, if for some reason your baby has to go to the NICU, you may not get to nurse him right away. Ask about the NICU policy for breast-feeding when you choose where you want to give birth. Other complications like eclampsia, pre-eclampsia, anemia, retained placenta, or bleeding after you give birth can reduce your supply and delay your ability to breastfeed. In these cases, your health is the first priority. If you can salvage breastfeeding afterward, great. If not, just making it through the birth is the real gift.

According to the CDC report from 2018, 31.9 percent of all births in the U.S. were by C-section. C-sections are sometimes planned and sometimes emergencies. Planned C-sections are when your baby is born in the hospital on a specific date that is scheduled by you and your obstetrician. It is sometimes planned for timing and convenience, but mostly because it is medically necessary. You could end up having a surprise C-section after starting out with a vaginal birth. This is called an unscheduled C-section, and there is always a medical reason for it. Emergency C-sections are different. They happen very quickly—sometimes within thirty total minutes—when there is a medical emergency, and your or your baby's life is at stake, or both of your lives.

C-sections are known to delay or even decrease overall rates of breastfeeding by 10 to 20 percent. But before taking that at face value, let's think about why it happens. Regardless of the type of C-section, they are all surgeries, which means you need anesthesia. Anesthesia could be a simple epidural, which numbs you below the waist. Epidurals don't really affect breast-feeding. But if you have full anesthesia (you are put completely to sleep), it will take some time for you to wake up, so you won't be able to nurse right away. The medications they give you to put you to sleep can also delay your hormones, like oxytocin and prolactin, so your milk supply can be delayed. Because your baby doesn't come through your birth canal, he isn't exposed to the bacteria from your vagina that help form his microbiome. Some doctors will coat him with it after a C-section, so ask about that beforehand. And often, the need for a C-section is because your baby can't be delivered vaginally. He may be breech or his head may be unable to fit through your pelvis. As we just learned, head shape affects breastfeeding too.

SKIN-TO-SKIN CONTACT

The immediate time after the delivery is a "sensitive period" that can promote your bonding to your baby. It happens best with skin-to-skin contact. Studies have shown that babies who get skin-to-skin immediately have a greater chance of breastfeeding.[4] Ideally, your baby will be laid prone on your bare chest. If your baby is full term, this simple connection will trigger a series of behaviors that help him find your breast. They are birth cry, relaxation, awakening and opening the eyes, activity (looking at you and your breast, rooting, hand-to-mouth movements, cooing), a second resting phase, crawling toward your nipple, touching and licking your nipple, suckling at the breast, and finally falling asleep. Some babies even massage their mom's breast with their hand.

DRUGS DURING AND AFTER LABOR

When you give birth, regardless of whether it's by C-section, you will have pain afterward and likely take some sort of pain-killer. One study showed that in the U.S., 83 percent of moms get pain meds regardless of the kind of delivery, and that pain medication can delay your milk production more than 23 percent of the time for at least three days.[5] Why does pain medication matter? For one thing, it can make you too sleepy to wake up and breastfeed. It can also dull the pain of a bad latch, so you may keep going even though something is wrong. If you are able to breastfeed, some of that pain medicine will get to your baby through your breastmilk. When it happens, he will be very sleepy and won't want to wake up to nurse. Over time, if he doesn't wake up to eat, he will lose weight.

Some drugs, like codeine, are transferred to your milk more than others, like hydrocodone. To be safe, take the smallest dose of pain medicine for less than three days if you can. You can take acetaminophen (Tylenol) and nonsteroidal anti-inflammatory drugs (NSAIDs; e.g., ibuprofen) instead of narcotics. But *always* avoid aspirin. Aspirin is hard for newborns to clear out of their bloodstream, so it can build up and become dangerous.

NICU AND PREMATURITY

Obviously, any reason your baby has to go to the NICU is concerning. Breastfeeding may be the last thing on your mind.

But even things that seem insurmountable, like cleft palate or open-heart surgery, don't have to make breastfeeding impossible. There are creative ways to nurse babies, so explore the possibilities before giving up.

If your baby is born early, you have to consider his due date. A few weeks early and his nursing reflexes may not be active yet. If he is born a month or more early, he may need to stay in the NICU and be fed in other ways at first. Don't despair. Your baby being in the NICU doesn't mean you won't have a breastfeeding relationship. You can still pump to keep your supply going and feed him bottled milk until you can start nursing.

Speaking of your supply, an early birth can also affect it. During pregnancy, you need time for your hormone prolactin to turn your breast tissue into milk-making factories. If your baby comes early, your breasts may not be ready to produce milk. You can have a delay in colostrum or milk while your hormones play catch-up.

TWINS AND MULTIPLE BIRTHS

There are a few things to think about when you want to breastfeed your newborn twins. In addition to the obvious need for more milk because there are two of them, twins often come before their due date. If they are premature (before 36 weeks), it may take some time until their reflexes are fully active. You will also need more time during the day to feed them. You can save time by nursing both babies simultaneously. This is called *tandem feeding*. You can also use tandem feeding as a way to compare your twins with each other. One baby may have a harder time nursing than the other or cause you pain. Having a real-time comparison can make problems more obvious early on so you can seek help sooner.

Challenges with feeding increase with every added baby, but if there is a will, there is usually a way. Should you be so blessed that you can make enough milk for more than two babies, more power to you. But be careful not to let your desire to breastfeed take time away from bonding with your babies in other ways. You will definitely need help!

LABOR AND DELIVERY NURSES AND LACTATION CONSULTANTS

If you give birth in the hospital, you will be visited by a rotating team of labor and delivery nurses. They will take care of you and your baby in every way, including checking your vitals and making sure your baby is fed and weighed. Labor and delivery nurses have such a huge number of responsibilities, it's not surprising that they aren't also experts in breastfeeding. Some have extra training, but most give advice based on either what they've personally experienced or what the plethora of moms they've worked with have gone through.

Although a diversity of experience is nice, it is also limited to what happens in the hospital. Nurses can be quite good at encouraging breastfeeding during your baby's first few days, but they don't see what happens when you get home. They know you need to rest after giving birth, so they may help by giving your baby formula, which may or may not fit your breastfeeding plan. They also have many other priorities, like making sure your baby is fed and caring for the other babies and moms on the floor, all with limited time. The bottom line is they need to get you ready for discharge as soon as possible. If your baby needs to be fed before your milk has come in or if you are struggling with the latch, they may not be able to help you in the hospital. They assume you will get help once you get home.

With more hospitals becoming Baby-Friendly, there is a good chance you will also be visited by a lactation consultant. The Baby-Friendly Hospital Initiative (BFHI) was launched by the World Health Organization (WHO) and the United Nations Children's Fund (UNICEF) in 1991 to help encourage breastfeeding worldwide. The nonprofit organization, Baby-Friendly USA (BFUSA), is the accrediting body of the BFHI, which helps hospitals incorporate the Ten Steps to Successful Breastfeeding and the International Code of Marketing Breastmilk substitutes. The BFHI has helped hospitals come a long way in encouraging education in breastfeeding during your postpartum time in the hospital to avoid incessant marketing from formula companies. In the United States, the number of births in Baby-Friendly hospitals has risen from 3 percent in 2007 to 28 percent in 2019. You can find a Baby-Friendly hospital by visiting the website www.babyfriendly usa.org. And with more birthing hospitals wanting to gain Baby-Friendly status, they are employing more lactation consultants.

If you are lucky enough to give birth in a hospital that has lactation consultants, take advantage of them. They can see you individually or a part of a group meetings. Like labor and delivery nurses, they have a whole floor of moms and babies to see, so you may not get much individual time. But any help is beneficial. Some even hold classes for outpatient moms to offer help after you leave the hospital, so make sure you ask about those.

While most lactation consultants employed by hospitals are IBCLCs, it doesn't mean they will give you a consistent message. Some have been around longer than others. If they work only in a hospital, they may be great for the first few days, but might have little experience in what happens once you get home. Some also work in pediatricians' offices, so you can follow up with them after you leave the hospital. When things are going as they should, lactation consultants are invaluable. They know the nuances of normal breastfeeding and encourage you to keep going when things seem insurmountable. But if something seems off, like you have pain beyond what you can handle or your baby wants to nurse all the time, make sure you dive deeper. If all you're getting is encouragement through suffering, don't assume you should just keep going. You need to figure out the underlying problem first.

Some lactation consultants will "diagnose" anatomic problems, such as tongue tie and lip tie. Although the diagnosis may be questionable, at least they are validating the fact that you are struggling. Many hospitals prohibit lactation consultants from diagnosing anything and won't allow them to give outside referrals to doctors or other healthcare practitioners who can help.

To further complicate the issue, obstetricians and pediatricians may not have the answers either. Your obstetrician will check you in the hospital to see how you are doing medically. Even though breasts are part of their specialty, it's unlikely they will ask you about breastfeeding. If they do, make sure to mention breast pain or nipple damage so they can check for an infection. Also, ask for a breast pump if you get engorged right away. They can order one for you to use while you are in the hospital. The hospital pediatrician also does rounds on all the newborns, doing assessments to make sure your baby is healthy. They may or may not ask about the quality of feedings, gas, or breast pain. Very rarely will they assess for tongue tie.

If you have problems nursing, your doctors may agree or disagree about whether you have a problem. They may also agree or disagree about the diagnosis and solution. Sadly, while everyone seems to be on board when it comes to basic health issues, every person who walks in the room will probably tell you something different about breastfeeding. When I see moms and babies in my office, they are often so confused about what and whom to believe. To them, I become yet another one of those people trying to convince them I'm right. All of us in the breastfeeding community are responsible for this confusion. If we can't get our story straight, how can we expect you to listen?

Although everyone has your well-being in mind, the biggest difference in advice is in the way we determine cause and effect. Part 3 of this book will go over red flags in detail to aid you in navigating through conflicting advice you get in the hospital. No matter what, if you believe something isn't right, look for answers.

HOME BIRTHS, MIDWIVES, AND DOULAS

If you have a home birth, your experience will be quite different from one in the hospital. You will have more control, for one. Often, home births are conducted by midwives, who are adept at spontaneous vaginal deliveries; i.e., natural childbirth. (Your baby can also be delivered by a midwife in the hospital.) As we know, these kinds of deliveries lend themselves to breastfeeding most. You will have more time to bond with your baby and not be subjected to hospital schedules. Your midwife may also have extra training in breastfeeding, so she can help you individually.

Many moms employ a doula to help with the delivery and early postpartum weeks. Doulas are a valuable source of support and information. They are trained companions who provide physical and emotional comfort and encouragement. They can also act as mediators in the hospital and at home to explain medical terms and procedures. Being trained as a doula doesn't automatically mean they have extra training in breastfeeding, but some do. Ask to be sure. They can also refer you to lactation consultants and doctors who work with breastfeeding babies should you need more help.

Baby's First Week

Now that the delivery is behind you, take a breath. After a deep inhale and exhale, get ready, because the real work is up ahead. The first twelve weeks after you give birth are just as important to your and your baby's well-being as the forty weeks of pregnancy. It is during this time that your baby adjusts to the world and you adjust to your new role as mom. Some cultures even refer to these weeks as the fourth trimester. During this sacred time, moms are given special diets and massages. They have organized help with the baby so they can sleep and don't overtax themselves. In this new experience for them, moms have community support. Raising a child takes a village. Unfortunately, that's not how it works in the United States.

In sharp contrast, as an American mom, you may find yourself completely alone when you take your baby home. Cast into the role of new mom, there is very little built-in support. Moms are encouraged and expected to "bounce back" quickly. Not only is this tragic, but it's also unrealistic. It takes time for you to settle into your new role, not to mention your new body and the new human you're caring for. You need a supportive spouse, a baby nurse or relative, and a babysitter or nanny to help with older siblings.

Having the right kind of support in your first weeks together is so important, especially when it comes to breast-feeding. Those first days at home can make or break your breastfeeding relationship (no pressure). Moms are at the greatest risk of giving up during the first week. Nearly every mom has concerns, especially when it comes to milk supply, pain, and the baby not being able to latch. The irony is that this is also the time you are least likely to have help.

When you do ask for help, make sure you get sound clinical guidance, not confusing advice. Don't assume that common problems are "normal" just because everyone tells you they are. As you learned in Chapter 2, if you are told to just "wait it out," you may miss a window of opportunity you can't make up later. The first week is a big transition time, so patterns may not be obvious right away.

In this chapter, we will talk about everything you need to know for the first week of nursing, putting everything we've learned thus far in context. We will go through what it should feel like, how to determine if your milk supply is coming in as it should, what you should be eating and drinking, and how you should be taking care of yourself. We will also discuss how much milk your baby needs and how often she should be nursing. You will learn which struggles are a normal part of the learning curve and when you need to call in outside help.

How Breastfeeding Should Feel

When your baby is born, she has all the reflexes she needs to nurse immediately. Your baby will root when she's hungry. This is an early cue, and one you should heed. It's better to start a feed when she turns her head to your chest and puts her fingers in her mouth than to wait for her to scream in hunger.

When your baby latches on correctly, it should feel good. And by good, I mean profoundly good. The physical touch of her mouth on your areola makes your brain release oxytocin. Oxytocin makes you feel love. It warms your heart and fills you with peace and bliss. Other than a little soreness from figuring out the initial latch, this whole process should be full of pleasant sensations.

You will notice right away if your baby can't gape widely enough. Babies are often called lazy when they don't gape, as though they have a choice. When babies can't gape, they may seem like they have "small" mouths, or they may purse their lips when they get to the breast. Sometimes babies who can't gape fall off and need to relatch over and over again. A small gape can also be quite painful for you. I call the nipple the "alarm" because it is the most sensitive part of your breast. If your nipple hurts when your baby latches on, the pain is an alarm that tells you something is wrong. Remember, the gape is a reflex. If your baby doesn't do it consistently in the first few days, it means she can't. She will not get better at it without intervention. And don't let anyone tell you otherwise!

Determining Your Milk Supply

Although it is hard to know exactly how much milk you are making, you will get used to using indirect ways to measure it. It seems scary at first, because you want to make sure you're making enough milk for your baby. But, thankfully, your baby comes preloaded with excess water weight for the first few days to help her out.

When it comes to supply, every woman is different. If things are going well, your breasts should look and feel bigger and fuller by the end of the first week. From Days 1 to 3, your breasts start making colostrum. That's the sticky, often yellowish early milk that has everything your baby needs for the first few days. Even though the amount of colostrum you make may not seem like much, it is enough to fill your baby's tiny stomach. By the end of the week your milk will turn into transitional milk, that in-between milk that's on its way to becoming mature breastmilk. You will also make more of it to fill your baby's growing stomach. Your breasts should get fuller. They will also leak milk when you hear your baby cry or touch her.

During the first few days, nursing should feel good, and that good feeling will help your brain release more prolactin. Remember that prolactin is especially important in the first few weeks because it turns your breast tissue into milk-making factories. The more prolactin you make early on, the better your chances of having a bigger supply down the road.

If for any reason your baby can't nurse in the first week, you can mimic this feeling on your own. You can use a warm, wet towel or hand stimulation. Gentle pumping can also be helpful. Similarly, if you are having a lot of pain when you nurse, it's better to stop and use hand expression or nipple stimulation with gentle pumping to give your supply a chance to come in until you take care of the underlying problem.

Your supply will vary throughout the day. Most moms have the most milk first thing in the morning because your brain makes more prolactin when you sleep. Similarly, your supply will tend to decrease into the evening, so your baby may want to nurse more often in the evenings.

Pumping and Hand Expressing

You may be confused about whether to pump during the first week. The answer is, it depends. Although I'm always a fan of having extra breastmilk in the fridge, it's not for everyone. You may have different goals and priorities, and supply is widely variable.

During the first week, most moms fall into one of four situations:

1. Your milk hasn't come in yet and there is nothing to pump.

2. Your milk is coming in and you want to nurse as much as possible.

3. Your milk is coming in and you want to store some bottles.

4. You have so much milk your baby can't drain your breasts fast enough.

Regardless of the situation, you can benefit from either pumping or hand stimulation. If your milk hasn't come in yet, hand stimulation and a silicone suction milk collector may be all you need. Sometimes moms can't get any milk out of their breasts with suction alone, so pumping with a motorized pump may be an exercise in futility. But don't discount the power of oxytocin. Whenever in doubt, stimulate your nipples with a warm, wet washcloth and try hand expression to get your hormones going.

Pressing or gently rubbing your nipples for a few seconds makes your brain release oxytocin and prolactin. If you follow that with hand pumping for two minutes, then change to a mechanical pump, it will mimic the way your baby nurses. It will also increase the fat content in your milk. If you do these things for the first three days after your baby is born, it can increase your supply and fat content for at least the first two months. If you suspect you have a low supply, start doing it right after you give birth. If your baby is older, and especially if he can't nurse well, you can do it every time you pump.

If your breasts fill up quickly this week, they can become engorged. Engorgement happens when your breasts get so full of milk and extra blood flow that the tubes that carry the milk get squeezed closed, preventing the milk from coming out. Hand expressing or pumping can be helpful and prevent a breast infection. It can at least relieve the pain and decompress your breasts enough so your baby can latch on. If you have a huge supply, you may be told not to pump by your pediatrician and/or lactation consultant. But remember, it's all about balance. If you are full, pump off enough to be comfortable. If your breasts fill up again quickly, read about how to manage a huge supply in Chapter 11.

Pumping is vital in the first week if, for whatever reason, your baby isn't nursing. You can't afford to leave your breasts full without emptying them, or you won't be able to lay down a good supply for the long run. A general rule is to pump from six to ten times a day for ten to fifteen minutes on each side (you can pump both at the same time). Prolonged pumping sessions are not necessary. You need to empty out your breasts as quickly and fully as possible, then give them time to fill up again. Don't miss this window of opportunity.

Diet and Hydration

Your body has a lot of recovering to do the first week, and you'll need more than just prenatal vitamins to do it. If you want to treat yourself with all your favorite foods, go for it, but don't go crazy. Although junk food can make your mouth happy, it won't make your body happy. Certain foods can help restore your body more quickly and support breastfeeding, so try to indulge in actual nutrition as well.

Iron is important for the obvious reason that you lose blood during the delivery. With a vaginal birth, you lose around 500 milliliters, or about a pint. With a C-section you could lose twice that amount, or a liter. Your blood is full of hemoglobin and hemoglobin is made from iron, so when you lose blood, you lose iron. Low iron can make you feel weak, tired, and depressed. You can take iron supplements, but they tend to cause constipation, which won't help your new hemorrhoids. Foods like lean red meat, spinach, lentils, beans, and fortified cereals are good sources of iron. Eating them with other foods that have vitamin C, like lemons and oranges, can help you better absorb the iron.

Calcium is especially important during pregnancy for your baby's bone development, among other things. You are her sole source of food when you're pregnant, so she will pull calcium from your body through her umbilical cord. If you aren't eating food with enough calcium or taking supplements, you may be low when you give birth. When the calcium runs low in your blood, it draws from your bones to make up for the difference. Breastfeeding creates another draw on your calcium. Over time this can lead to bone loss and potentially osteoporosis, fragile bones that can break easily. Although you can increase your calcium with obvious things, like dairy, your body actually absorbs it more easily from plants, such as broccoli and other green leafy vegetables. Sardines or canned fish with bones, soybeans, tofu, and fortified cereals and juices are also good sources of calcium.

You need protein to help heal your body from the trauma of childbirth. Whether you had a quick vaginal birth or a more complex C-section, your body needs a variety of proteins to help you heal. Protein breaks down into amino acids, which help your body make hormones, like serotonin, that help guard you against postpartum depression. Breastfeeding increases your need for protein even more—by 25 grams a day. If you're a meat eater, stick with lean cuts of chicken, turkey, and beef.

There are also plant-based protein sources, like peas or pea powder, tofu and tempeh, quinoa, and beans. Nuts have protein, but they are mostly fat, so eat them sparingly.

When you produce breastmilk, you also need more fluids and calories. Drink ten to twelve glasses of water a day and avoid drinks that can dehydrate you, like caffeinated teas and coffee. Increase your food intake by about 500 calories a day. That's a couple of snacks or an extra-small meal. Omega-3 fatty acids, especially DHA, are good for your baby's brain development. You can take supplements or eat fatty fish, but be careful of eating fish that can be contaminated with mercury. Salmon, herring, mackerel, sardines, and caviar are good choices.

Although we talk about food and diet a lot, we often forget to mention your digestion and bowels. The dramatic shift in your hormones can cause constipation or loose bowels. All the pushing from the delivery and extra weight from the pregnancy can cause hemorrhoids. Change in bowel movements and hemorrhoids aren't the best combination. Add to them pain from a healing episiotomy, and you have a recipe for very uncomfortable trips to the bathroom.

Increasing the fiber in your diet through leafy greens, blueberries, and grains will help soften your stool naturally. Probiotics can also be helpful. Fennel and fenugreek can help with excess gas, and also increase your milk supply. Tums are helpful for heartburn and double as a calcium supplement.

Self-Care

The first week after you give birth, your body may feel completely foreign. Between the surprise uterine cramping, hot flashes from hormones readjusting, swollen legs and feet from fluid shifts during pregnancy, sore muscles from the actual birth, and bleeding after delivery, you will swear your body has been inhabited by an alien. In these first days, while your body settles into its new normal, you need to make yourself as much of a priority as your new baby. It may seem impossible, but you need rest. Ideally, you will have help so you aren't doing it all yourself. Before you give birth, create a postpartum plan, compiling a list of family, friends, and professionals to help, so you know who you can rely on. You can do some planning in advance, like stocking the kitchen with groceries and writing lists so others can shop for you after you get home. Ask for help with grocery shopping, housecleaning, and laundry. You can also research postpartum support groups, breastfeeding groups, and partners for walks. Take time to check out these groups before you give birth, so you have familiar faces when you introduce your baby.

There are many ways you can nurture yourself through this first week. Yoga, in the form of simple pelvic stretching, is safe in the first week. Avoid anything strenuous. Sitz baths, where you soak your perineum in a bath or basin of warm water, are a godsend. You can make a sitz bath by adding bicarbonate or Epsom salts to the water. Drugstores sell kits, but the hospital can also give you one to take home.

Massage is an often-overlooked but wonderful addition to postpartum care. Safe human touch makes your brain release oxytocin, and massage does the same thing. It can help regulate out-of-whack hormones so you can get better sleep and have better milk production. It also helps reduce body swelling and inflammation and quells anxiety and depression. If you had a vaginal birth, you can have a massage within the first week. For C-section moms, you should wait to lie face-forward until your incision heals. No matter how you give birth, you can still have your shoulders rubbed. Even if you don't get a professional massage, ask your partner to rub your feet or hands. Good touch is your friend in these first few weeks.

Breastfeeding may take up a lot of your time, but that time should feel like a reward for carrying your baby for forty weeks. It should be part of your healing and not an added stress to get in the way of bonding with your baby. Remember: Breastfeeding helps you bond only if the net result is positive. If you nurse through toe-curling pain and cry at the thought of your baby's mouth on your breast, breastfeeding can do more damage than not breastfeeding at all. Don't suffer in silence. Do as much as you can in this first week to nurture yourself.

How Much Milk Your Baby Needs in Week 1

At birth, your baby is waterlogged from swimming around in amniotic fluid for nine months. This extra fluid gives her some protection from dehydration while your milk comes in. It is normal for her to lose 7 to 10 percent of her birth weight during the first three to seven days as her body releases this excess fluid. The low point will be Day 4, but her weight should turn around after that.

In the first few days, you make only colostrum, but it's just the right amount to fit in her tiny stomach. Her needs and the size of her stomach are synced up with your milk supply, so her stomach grows as your supply does. When she is born, her stomach is the size of an olive and can hold 5 to 7 milliliters (about a teaspoon) at each feeding. On the first day, she will need to eat a total of 20 to 40 milliliters (5 to 8 teaspoons) divided up into eight to ten feedings. By Day 3, her stomach grows to the size of a Ping-Pong ball. She can eat 22 to 27 milliliters per feeding (about an ounce) for a total of 10 to 19 ounces a day. By the end of the first week, her stomach will grow to the size of a lime, and she will be able to eat 40 to 60 milliliters per feeding (1.5 to 2.0 ounces) and a total of 14 to 22 ounces a day.

If you bottle-feed her at all this week, make sure to use a Level 1 nipple for newborns. These nipples, regardless of brand, have one hole for the milk to come through, so your baby doesn't get too much flow. Also, keep in mind that when you nurse, your baby gets a steady flow of milk that is sugary foremilk first, followed by fatty hindmilk. When the fatty hindmilk reaches her small intestine, her brain releases a hormone called *cholecystokinin (CCK)*. CCK has many effects, including helping with digestion and letting your baby know she is full so she stops eating and goes to sleep.[1]

CCK is released in two ways. When your baby starts sucking, a little bit is released. It doesn't matter what she sucks on, whether it's your breast or a pacifier. That little bit of CCK fades away after ten minutes. After thirty to sixty minutes of active nursing, the fat from your milk should have finally made its way to her small intestine, triggering another, bigger release of CCK. This big release of CCK makes your baby so sleepy, she should stay asleep for two to three hours.

The younger your baby, especially when she is really tiny, the more CCK she has floating around all the time. This is why babies tend to sleep a lot when they are first born. Similarly, if your baby is nursing and not getting enough milk, she will fall asleep quickly but wake up hungry after a few minutes. If the milk fat from your hindmilk doesn't make it to her small intestine, a second release of CCK won't be triggered to help her stay asleep longer. If you have a big supply and your baby is only getting the sugary foremilk, the same thing can happen. If you give your baby pumped milk or formula, the fatty parts are mixed in, so your baby doesn't have the same timing of cues to tell her she's full. That's why paced bottle-feeding is important. Otherwise, it is very easy to overfeed a baby. It's also why breastfed babies are better at self-regulating. Their hormones are designed that way.

Without a "full" sensor, your baby may eat far more than her stomach can hold at one time. Try to stay within the guidelines of what she needs when you bottle-feed and don't just feed her as much as she will take.

Timing of Nursing

As early as the first week, your baby will start to make associations between her time at your breast and how satisfied she is.

Although the number of times a day you nurse, how well your baby empties your breasts, and how long it takes her to nurse will vary the most during the first week, you will notice a pattern early on. This pattern is important. The more pleasant and efficient your nursing experience during this week, the more milk-making factories and prolactin receptors you make. Even though there is a certain amount of flexibility, this early time sets the stage for your whole nursing relationship.

Your baby is born with a set of reflexes that let you know when she's hungry. She will root and put her hand to her mouth or turn her head to your breast. It's best to follow these early cues rather than wait for her to cry or get frantic. Once your baby is screaming, it's harder to tell what she needs. Sudden crying may mean it's been too long since she's eaten and she's starving. But it may mean something completely different, especially if you just fed her. It could be that she's in pain from gas or colic or has a dirty diaper. If your baby is frantic, it's best to calm her down, check her diaper, or try to burp her before attempting a latch.

Once your baby is latched on and nursing feels good, certain patterns will develop. Your baby may not eat on a regular schedule, but she should nurse, on average, for ten to fifteen minutes on each breast, every two to two and a half hours, or eight to ten times a day. Usually babies get more milk in the early mornings, when your supply is greatest, and less as the day goes on. Around early afternoon, they can nurse more often, which is called *cluster feeding*.

Although cluster feeding is common, it isn't always normal and shouldn't be ignored. If your baby is attached to your breast for hours, falls asleep, and cries when you take her off, this isn't typical cluster feeding. It means she may not be getting enough milk from you. One way to test how much she is getting is to pump after you've nursed for ten to fifteen minutes on each side. If you have milk left, especially if her latch is painful, she may not be transferring milk out of you. Another test is to offer her a bottle after she nurses for ten to fifteen minutes. If she gobbles it up, either you aren't producing enough or she isn't transferring it out. See Chapter 12 for guidance.

What Goes in Must Come Out

Babies are remarkably good at following this rule. Starting at Day 1, her number of stools and wet diapers will increase each day. During the first twenty-four hours, between releasing what she takes in and the extra fluid she is born with, this usually means one wet diaper and one black, tarry stool. The tarry stool means her *meconium,* the waste she makes in the womb, is passing. By Day 4 she should make four stools and four wet diapers. By the end of week one, she should make six to seven wet diapers and at least four stools a day.

The color and amount of her wet and dirty diapers is also important. Not all wet diapers are the same, but they should each have at least 3 tablespoons (45 mL). Depending on the kind of diapers you use, the very absorbent, disposable ones can hold more urine. This makes it harder to tell how much she is wetting, so you might want to get a sense of it by practicing with different amounts of water. Her urine should be clear to light yellow. If she is dehydrated, she will make orange *crystals* from concentrated urate. Her stools should look green by Day 4, and, by the end of the week, change to yellow or yellowish brown. This color change means her bowels are working and her gut flora is developing nicely.

7

Weeks 2 to 4

The second to fourth week is the time with the most moving parts. Things can change on a daily basis, so get ready. Just when you start to have a rhythm, something new may pop up to keep you on your toes. To help make these weeks go more smoothly, this chapter will build on what we've already learned from Chapter 6. You will learn how nursing should ideally progress so you can identify budding problems before they blossom into bigger ones. I will describe how to handle your baby's rapidly increasing needs and how your supply increases to meet his needs. You will also learn how long and how often you should nurse to make sure your baby has the expected output and weight gain.

Remember, breastfeeding is complicated and individual. It is not one size fits all. The same set of circumstances can be perfect for one mom-and-baby dyad and not so great for another. In this section, I will describe normal, but keep in mind that normal is more of a reference point. There are variations in normal, but if you fall far outside its range, don't assume everything will work itself out. First, let's talk about your supply.

How to Determine Your Milk Supply in Weeks 2 to 4

Let's be honest: figuring out your supply is hard for a lot of reasons. There is no way to do it directly. You can't see inside your breasts to measure how much milk is in there. Your supply also changes on a daily basis and fluctuates throughout the day. In all honesty, you may never know your true supply.

This not knowing is as frustrating as it is anxiety-provoking. All moms worry about supply. Moms are so concerned about not making enough milk, it is one of the top three reasons they stop breastfeeding during the first month. When your only assurance is encouragement to keep going, you could be sadly disappointed. So how can you feel more confident that you have enough milk? By understanding how your supply works and using other clues to fill in the gaps. Then and only then can you sit back and trust.

Milk supply is not just one measurement. It is a complicated combination of the following three things:

1. Storage capacity: how much you can store at once

2. Rate of production: how fast your breasts make milk

3. Rate of flow: how fast the milk comes out

On the one hand, it's impossible to get exact measures. On the other, because there are so many variables, you can do different things to change your supply. We will talk more about it in Chapter 11.

Because you can't test these measurements out individually, we tend to rely on more subjective comparisons: things we can see and feel. These comparisons can be helpful, but if you have no frame of reference, they are useless. They are also constantly changing. If you're a first-time mom, you may feel even more in the dark because you don't have another breastfeeding experience to compare to.

Here is a list of the most common ways moms are told to test their supply, explained so you understand them in context:

1. *Your breasts should be firmer and larger than they were before pregnancy.*

   It seems easy enough to tell if your breasts are firmer and larger, but how firm and how large should they be? During the first week, most moms get *engorged* at some point. Engorgement is when your breasts fill up with milk and increased blood flow. Sometimes they get so full, milk can't come out of the ducts and your breasts hurt from the pressure. This is normal for a few days, but if it persists for longer, you have to address it beyond just nursing and/or pumping. The ideal fullness and firmness are somewhere between "bigger than before" and engorged. Remember, size and firmness don't really tell you how much milk is inside. They just give you a hint that things are moving in the right direction. If by the second week your breasts don't seem much different than before pregnancy, you may be a low producer. Conversely, if they are so full, they feel like they are going to explode, you may have to adjust how and when you empty them.

2. *Your baby should seem satisfied after you nurse him.*

During the first month, your baby's needs change on a daily basis. Your supply is also changing to meet his needs. If everything is going well, he should be able to get everything he needs from you. But summing up that whole supply-and-demand relationship into the word *satisfied* is confusing. Is he satisfied if he falls asleep often in the middle of nursing? Does he pass out because he's full or too exhausted from trying? Does *satisfied* mean he smiles and burps and stays up? When he is less than a month old, his cues are different than when he's older. During this early time, a more complete way to interpret whether he is satisfied is this: After nursing for ten to fifteen minutes on each breast with a wide gape, a deep latch, active nursing, and pleasant sensations for you, your baby should fall asleep and stay sleeping for at least two hours and not wake up a few minutes later crying from hunger or gas. You should notice him swallowing and hear him gulping nearly every time he sucks.

3. *Your breasts should get softer after you nurse.*

If your breasts are firm or engorged, it will be harder for your baby to latch on and get a good seal. Imagine trying to fit your mouth around an orange. That being said, once your baby transfers out some milk, your breast should soften and become more moldable. You should notice this softening pretty quickly, especially after your first letdown. After ten minutes, there should be a noticeable difference, as though you squeezed water out of a sponge. If it takes more than thirty minutes for your breasts to soften, or if you don't notice much of a change, either you make a huge amount of milk or your baby isn't able to transfer it out.

4. *Your breasts should leak milk.*

When you touch your baby or hear him cry, your brain releases oxytocin. Oxytocin gets your milk flowing. While most moms leak milk pretty early on, the leakage alone doesn't guarantee that you have a good supply. It just tells you your hormones are working. If you don't have leakage, check for other things like engorgement and fullness to make sure your supply is coming in as it should.

5. *You should get X amount of milk when you pump.*

Pumping is a funny thing. Breast pumps are machines that are only able to pull out milk using a vacuum. Some moms need the extra push from oxytocin to empty their breasts. Others need the compression from the baby's mouth. The problem is, you don't know what you don't know. If this is your first baby, you may not know how your lactating breasts work. Even if your breasts are firmer and harder than before, you may only be able to pump out a few drops. Also, when, how often, and how long you pump matters. If you pump first thing in the morning after sleeping for four hours, you will likely pump out more than if you pump every two hours. Pumping can give you a sense of how much milk you produce at any given time, but it doesn't necessarily reflect your total milk supply.

How Much Milk You Should Be Making in Weeks 2 to 4

No matter what you've been told, all moms make differing amounts of milk. Think of milk supply as a spectrum. Some moms make very little and will never have a full supply. Most moms make an average amount. Some make so much it's almost too much. During the first month, you will get a sense of where you fall in the spectrum. But keep in mind, your supply is also based on your baby's ability to transfer out your milk. If your baby nurses for weeks and never empties your breasts, your supply will go down over time and never be what it could have been.

For an average milk producer, from Weeks 1 to 4, your supply should grow from around 14 ounces a day to 28 to 32 ounces a day. For comparison, 14 ounces is about $1^3/_4$ measuring cups, and 28 to 32 ounces is $3^1/_2$ to 4 cups. At the end of the first month, most moms make 1,100 milliliters, or just over 4 cups of milk per day, which is where it will usually stay.

After the first month, it is much harder to increase your supply, so it's important to keep track of what you're producing early on and do your best to keep it going. If you let this early time pass, you may miss your biggest window of opportunity for a long-term milk supply.

As a reminder from Chapter 6, prolactin levels are very high in your bloodstream for the first seven to ten days. After that, the amount of prolactin your brain releases sharply decreases. This means that there will be a smaller amount of prolactin to stimulate your breasts to make milk. If you did a good job emptying your breasts regularly during the first week, you should be in a good place now. Your breasts should have a lot of prolactin receptors on their milk-making factories, so they will be really sensitive to that small amount of prolactin. If you weren't able to remove milk regularly or if you had a lot of pain during the first seven to ten days, you may not have made as many milk-making factories. The tiny bit of prolactin in your bloodstream won't turn on as much milk production, so your storage capacity will be lower. You may have to nurse more often to compensate, or you may inadvertently end up with a lower total milk supply.

Timing of Milk Removal

From Day 10 on, your supply becomes even more dependent on the way your breasts are emptied.

As we discussed in Chapter 3, this is because your breasts make feedback inhibitor of lactation (FIL) at the same rate they make milk. As FIL fills your breasts, the milk-making factories stop making milk. The fuller your breasts, the more FIL there is floating around, the less prolactin can stimulate milk production, and the less milk you make. When FIL is removed—which happens only when your milk is removed—more milk can be produced. The amount of milk you make also depends on how quickly you remove FIL. If you remove milk slowly, your breasts will fill up slowly. If you remove it quickly, they will fill up quickly. Similarly, if you always have milk in your breasts, they will make less milk. If you empty them out completely, they are free to make enough milk to fill up again. If you want to maximize your supply early on, it's best to empty your breasts quickly (ten to fifteen minutes on each side) and completely (they should feel very soft and empty), then wait two hours for them to fill up again, and repeat.

It is possible that one reason some women have a huge supply is that they don't make much FIL. No one has studied this, but it is highly likely. Some moms just keep making milk without a stopgap. Other moms may make too much FIL, so their breasts are very sensitive to how they are emptied.

It may seem that the only way you can have a big supply is if you have a huge storage capacity, but that's not necessarily true. A mom may have a small storage capacity but make milk quickly. If she nurses more frequently, she can give her baby the same amount of milk as a mom who has a normal supply. Conversely, if a mom has a big storage capacity or fast letdown, her baby may nurse for a short amount of time and still get a lot of milk.

There are so many factors that affect supply, and everyone is different, so pay attention to how your body works. Your ability to produce milk is truly the most variable part of breastfeeding.

Your Baby's Growing Needs

By Weeks 2 to 3, your baby's stomach can hold approximately 60 to 90 milliliters (2 to 3 oz) at each feeding, with a total of 600 to 750 milliliters (20 to 25 oz) per day. His stomach is the size of a large egg or kiwi fruit, so it can hold a quarter to a third of a measuring cup of milk at a time. By Week 4, your baby's needs increase to 90 to 120 milliliters (3 to 4 oz) per feeding, and 750 to 1050 milliliters per day (25 to 35 oz). This is about half a measuring cup of milk at a time.

When you breastfeed, just like it's impossible to know your exact milk supply, there is no way to measure exactly how much milk your baby is getting. Some lactation consultants or pediatricians weigh babies on an infant scale before and after nursing. Even that is only a rough measure. Unless you feed your baby with a bottle, you have to rely on subjective measures from your baby to make sure he is getting enough.

If you have a normal supply, after nursing for about ten to fifteen minutes on each side, your baby should fall asleep for two to three hours. He should root when he's hungry, put his hands to his mouth, and nurse calmly. You should hear gulping when he eats and see him swallow with every one to two sucks. He should also be able to stay latched on to you without slipping off and crying. If he wakes up screaming or sleeps for only a few minutes and then wakes up hungry and flustered, he is probably not getting enough milk.

By the end of the first month, your baby will need the same volume of milk that he needs for the duration of nursing, no matter how long you decide to nurse.

Timing and Frequency of Feeding

Your total milk supply affects how often and how long your baby nurses. If you have a low or high supply, your baby will nurse differently than if you have an average supply. Assuming you have an average supply and that your baby is able to gape and latch normally, he should nurse every two to three hours for ten to fifteen minutes on each side, which means you should be feeding him about eight times a day by the end of the first month. Let's discuss where these numbers come from.

Your letdown starts thirty to forty-five seconds after you start nursing. Each letdown lasts forty-five seconds to three and a half minutes and can happen up to four times in a session, depending on how long you nurse. With the first letdown, after one to four minutes, half the milk in your breasts is pushed out. Say you have two more letdowns that happen a few minutes apart. After roughly ten minutes, most of the milk in your breasts should be emptied. If you nurse for longer—say, twenty to thirty minutes—the law of diminishing returns rears its ugly head. Sometimes babies graze or take breaks during a feeding, which is fine, but they shouldn't spend most of the session sleeping. The ten to fifteen minutes should be active nursing. Your baby fast asleep with your nipple in his mouth doesn't count.

Now that we've established ideal, let's talk about reality. Over the course of the day, your baby's feeding patterns will vary. Although current recommendations in the breastfeeding community is baby-led feeding, merely following your baby's cues doesn't guarantee successful nursing. You have to also make sure your baby is gaping normally, latching on well, and transferring out milk, and you have to know your supply so you can accurately interpret what's happening. Your baby's behavior is important, because it's another way to tell if things are going well.

For example, if your baby is hungry all the time or nurses every hour, he is either not getting enough or working really hard to get what he is getting. This may or may not correlate with breast pain, milk supply, or weight gain, but it usually does. Conversely, if you have a high milk supply but your baby has a poor latch and can't transfer milk well, he may compensate by nursing all the time and sleeping through feedings. He may, in fact, gain weight, but he is working too hard. It's like he is trying to suck milk out of a straw with a hole in it.

Your Baby's Weight Gain and Output

There are a lot of ways to look at weight gain and different ways to measure it. After the first week, your baby should follow these patterns.

- $2/3$ to 1 ounce (19 to 28 g) a day
- 4 to 7 ounces ($1/4$ to $1/2$ lb, or 112 to 200 g) a week
- 32 ounces (2 lbs, or 0.9 kg) a month

Your baby should grow 0.5 to 1 inch (about 1.5 to 2.5 cm) by the end of the first month. Growth spurts happen at two to three weeks, six weeks, and three months.

Five to six wet diapers every twenty-four hours is the expectation. Each diaper should have about 3 tablespoons (or 45 mL) of wetness in them. You might want test what that feels like by pouring water in the diapers you plan to use. Most babies have four poopy diapers a day for the first four to six weeks, but it drops down to once a day or less after that. Breastfed babies have stool that is soft and runny.

How to Use Pumping and Bottle Feeding

A whole book could be written on how and when to pump, especially if you have decided to pump and not nurse. Breast-feeding doesn't always mean your baby has to get the milk out himself. Pumping and bottle-feeding is another way to give your baby breastmilk, and it shouldn't be discounted. Similarly, just because you are breastfeeding, it doesn't mean you have to nurse your baby every time you feed him. You need to take breaks and let others help.

During the first month, pumping can be a blessing, even if you plan to exclusively nurse. Here are instances where it can be helpful:

1. If your baby can't or won't empty your breasts, pumping can get that last bit out to build up your supply or keep it going.

2. You can pump and store milk so you can take a break.

3. Pumping off the first bit of milk can make your breasts softer when they are engorged or very full, so your baby can latch on more easily.

Make sure you have a well-fitting flange so you don't traumatize your nipples. You can even warm the flanges or use warm, wet towels to help stimulate your letdown before you pump. Looking at a picture of your baby or hearing him cry or coo also works. You can enlist your partner's help in this too. Remember that person?

When bottle-feeding, use a Level 1 nipple. It has only one

hole in it to slow the flow. There are countless nipples and bottles that promise to help with things like gas and colic. Some say they mimic the breast, but they can't. They are all made of silicone or plastic, and the nipples feel nothing like your breasts. They are also not the shape your areola takes when your baby is latched on. If your baby has a hard time eating from a bottle or milk leaks out the sides, check his mouth for a high arched palate (see Chapter 12). Gas and colic usually happen as a result of your baby swallowing too much air because of this anatomy. None of these bottle nipples help with that, so don't waste your money buying all the different kinds.

Pillows, Positioning, and PT

There are many breastfeeding positions. I explained my favorite position for learning how to latch your baby on in Chapter 4—the cross-cradle. Here are other positions you may want to try. This list is far from exhaustive.

Figure 1: Cradle hold

Figure 2: Football hold

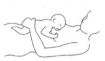

Figure 3: Laid-back hold

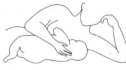

Figure 4: Side-lying hold

Figure 5: Upright hold

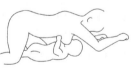

Figure 6: Dangle feeding

1. *Cradle hold*

   This is the classic breastfeeding position. You sit upright and hold your baby on his side with his tummy against your chest. The difference between this hold and the cross-cradle is where you put your arms. In this position, the same side arm as your breast is under your baby's head, and your other arm is around his legs. In these early weeks, it's hard to hold your baby this way without using pillows that prop him up and support your arms and back. You also aren't supporting your breast, so it's up to your baby to support his weight and keep himself latched on his own. This hold can be challenging or impossible if your baby has a restricted gape.

2. *Football hold*

   This very popular hold starts with sitting with your baby perpendicular to your breast. His body should be tucked along your side with his head near your breast and his feet behind you. You'll need to support his whole body with a pillow while he is small. It should support his head as he gets bigger. This position is good early on because it provides a lot of support and helps him feel safe. You also get to see his face more easily, and you have more control over his head. This position is great if you have twins or when you are recovering from a C-section.

3. *Laid-back hold*

   This is often the first way moms try to nurse in the delivery room. You lean back and latch your baby on, facing you, while he is on top. You don't have to lie completely flat. Lying against a pillow or cushion gives you the best angle.

Your baby can be either lengthwise or across your chest. This position works really well for newborns, because there is so much skin-to-skin contact. It is also good if you have a forceful letdown or huge supply. It gives your baby the chance to nurse against gravity without getting waterboarded.

4. *Side-lying hold*

This could turn into your favorite overnight position, especially if you are a fan of co-sleeping. It may even make you a fan of co-sleeping. You and your baby lie on your sides, facing each other, and you prop yourself up with your arm. It doesn't provide much support, but it works well if your baby has an easy latch.

5. *Upright hold*

In this position, you sit upright, against a pillow or backed chair, and your baby sits on your thigh facing you. This won't work as easily for a newborn, but as your baby gets older, he will have more head and neck control. This position is helpful if your baby has gas, colic, or low muscle tone. It is also good if you have a big supply.

6. *Dangle feeding*

This is not a position I would recommend on a regular basis, but it's great if you have engorgement or are recovering from mastitis. Some believe it even helps unclog blocked ducts. In this position, your baby lies on his back, and you crouch over him on all fours, latching him on to your dangling breast. You can use pillows to prop yourself up and support your knees.

In these early days, while you are figuring everything out, all the positioning and holding your breasts and your baby's head can get exhausting. You will feel it in your shoulders, neck, back, and arms, even if you're doing everything right. Just like the first week, massage, and even physical therapy, can be helpful in Weeks 2 to 4.

Supplementing with Formula

Obviously, this is a book about breastfeeding. But even if things are going perfectly in that respect, there may be times you need or want to use formula. Choose a kind that is supplemented with DHA/ARA. If your baby is reacting to it with a rash or excess gas, try a hypoallergenic formula made with amino acids instead of cow or soy milk. Although it is marketed within an inch of its life, and as moms we are trying to wean from our dependence on it, there will be times you need it. You could need it early on, before your milk comes in. Or later, when you pump and dump because you had to have ALL those glasses of wine. No matter how you feed your baby, you have to feed your baby. Reaching for a bottle of Similac does not make you a failure. Remember that breastfeeding is supposed to be your reward for carrying your baby through the pregnancy and giving birth. It should be another way to bond with him, but it's not the only way. Breastfeeding is not all or none. You can nurse and bottle-feed and formula-feed. Some days, you will feel lucky to have options.

8

Weeks 5 to 12 and Beyond

Congratulations! You've made it to Week 5! If you're feeling like a pro, you should. You've earned it. You made it through the first month with a whole new understanding of the way you and your baby work together. Even though you may be tired, the results are worth it. You may have even picked up a couple of new nursing positions or figured out how to pump while you eat.

Here's more good news: Moving forward, things should get easier. Your hard work in the first month is finally going to pay off. Your baby should fall into a more regular nursing routine and become more efficient as she gets bigger. Your breasts should start to make sense, making it easier to guess your supply. As time goes on, you should spend less time nursing and be able to do it without needing all the pillows and props. Those promises of the benefits of breastfeeding will finally be real.

In this chapter, I will explain how you should adjust your nursing schedule as your baby becomes more efficient. We will also discuss your baby's expected weight gain and how your supply and breasts may change. We will talk about pumping, bottles, and how to store and thaw milk.

If you've been following along in this book as you go, hopefully you've been able to catch problems as they arise. If you are just reading it now after nursing for a couple of months, you will see how things should be going. Things may have started out fine but seem to be headed in the wrong direction. If so, read this chapter, then jump ahead to Part 3 to help you understand what's gone wrong and options for fixing it.

Your Milk Supply

Around Week 5, you start to really get a sense of your supply. If the first month went smoothly, from Week 5 onward, your total milk supply should remain about the same at 1,100 milliliters, or $4\frac{1}{2}$ cups, or 32 ounces a day. This is an average, of course, and you may make more or less than this. I hesitate to use the terms *low supply* and *oversupply* if you fall outside this range. Supply is more of a spectrum than a discrete amount, and it's not all or none (PICTURE 6). Breastfeeding is a supply-and-demand thing. Your supply is customized to your baby, or babies, if you're feeding more than one at a time. Even if you have to supplement with formula, you can still breastfeed. Should you be an abundant producer, you can freeze the extra or donate it to a milk bank.

Sometimes a huge supply can mask underlying problems. Things may have seemed okay at first, but around Weeks 6 to 10 your supply starts to change. Your once full breasts that leaked now only have drips. When you pump, you get a lot less than you used to. Your baby may have gained a lot of weight at first, but now she cries after a few minutes and chokes on milk. She may have gas or want to eat all the time. Your pain may have subsided, and your nipples may have healed, but "out of nowhere" they start to hurt again. This is usually because your baby is having trouble transferring milk. Your once big supply covered up the problem, but after six to ten weeks, they change. Your baby has to pull out the milk or she won't get as much. You have to address the underlying problem. See Chapter 12 for help.

How Your Breasts Change

After the first month, your breasts should continue to feel full and firm. They should have the same storage capacity and milk production at six months as they do at one month. You will still make a consistent amount of milk as long as you keep emptying them fully and regularly. Prolactin is at a minimum now, so it gets released in tiny spurts after each time you nurse. But that little bit is enough to stimulate your breasts to fill up for the next feeding.

FIL is also in full force, preventing you from making too much milk and keeping your supply in check. To maintain your supply, you have to keep emptying your breasts. You shouldn't have to nurse every two hours, like when your baby was under a month old, but if you take a long time to empty your breasts, say forty-five minutes to an hour, or go for more than a few hours without emptying them, your supply will eventually decrease. It may not seem obvious at first, but after a few weeks or months, you will notice less milk. You may also get plugged ducts or bouts of mastitis.

From one month on, the goal is to keep your breasts making a steady supply for as long as you decide to breastfeed, whether it's two months or twenty-two months. If your supply matches your baby's needs, it's easy to keep track. But pay attention to slow or sudden changes in your breasts because they may be trying to alert you to a problem you may have missed.

After six months, your breasts will change again. They usually soften and shrink a little. By fifteen months, they may even get to their pre-pregnancy size. But don't let their smallness fool you. Even after a year, your breasts can produce a substantial amount of milk. They may look like regular breasts, but they will have a lot more milk-making factories and be able to produce milk more efficiently.

Amount of Milk Your Baby Needs

From one to six months, your baby still needs only 32 ounces of milk a day, but, because her stomach grows as she gets older, she can take in more volume with each feeding. At one month, her stomach can hold about 3 to 4 ounces at a time, about the same volume as an egg or one-third to one-half of a measuring cup. By six months, her stomach is the size of a large grapefruit, so it can hold about 6 ounces, or $^3/_4$ of a cup, at a time. By one year, it can hold about 2 cups at a time. After that it grows steadily until adulthood, when the average stomach size reaches 4 cups or the size of a small melon.

The Timing of Nursing

As your baby gets bigger, she should take less time at the breast to get the same amount of milk. This is because her jaw, head, and neck muscles get stronger as she gets older. She will have better head control so she can hold your breast in her mouth with less help. She will pause less, have longer suck bursts, and be able to create a stronger vacuum suction to pull milk out more quickly and forcefully.

Because babies become more efficient during the first four months, the timing changes. You may still nurse for ten to fifteen minutes at each session, but the time between sessions will increase so you can nurse less often. By six weeks your baby should be able to go three hours between feeds. By ten to twelve weeks she will probably nurse every four hours and/or snack on and off. The same is true by six months, but each time she feeds, she will get more milk to fill her growing stomach.

As your baby gets older, the time she spends nursing will also become more variable. At three months, she may nurse for five minutes and get the same amount she got in fifteen minutes when she was three weeks. As she gets older, she will be more aware of her surroundings and get distracted. As she gets closer to ten weeks, variable nursing times are expected, but remember to keep looking at the big picture. Her breastfeeding sessions should still be shorter and less often overall. If your ten-week-old still wants to nurse every two hours or takes thirty minutes to nurse, she's probably not getting enough milk. Conversely, she may be so good at pulling out milk, she can down four ounces in five minutes. How will you know she's getting enough milk? By keeping track of her weight gain.

Your Baby's Weight Gain

From one to four months, your baby should gain 1.5 to 2 pounds each month and grow at a rate of 1 to 1.5 inches a month. She will gain fat as well as muscle. That chubby face and the rolls of fat around her wrists will get bigger the first few months, and then she will start to lean out by five to six months. By six months, your baby should double her birth weight. By twelve months, she will have tripled it. Over the first year she will grow 9 to 11 inches. Her growth is the fastest over the first six months, and then it slows down in the second half of his first year.

Another way to look at it is this:

WEIGHT CHANGES IN BABY OVER THE FIRST YEAR

- Birth to 4 days: 7 to 10 percent loss of birth weight
- 4 days to 4 months: gain of 2 pounds per month (7 to 8 oz, or 200 to 225 g per week)
- 4 to 6 months: gain of 1 pound per month (4 to 5 oz, or 113 to 142 g per week)
- 6 to 12 months: gain of $3/4$ pound per month (3 to 4 oz, or 85 to 113 g per week)

Breastmilk- and formula-fed babies grow at about the same rate for the first three months. From four to six months, breastfed babies gain weight more slowly than their formula-fed friends, but their length and head circumference grow at the same rate. After six months, breastfed babies gain about a pound less a month. If you are feeding your baby both breastmilk and formula, the difference will be less noticeable. Don't worry about this difference in weight. Although all kinds of studies show that breastfed babies are less prone to obesity, illness, and so on, this is true for populations of babies. It's harder to make sense of these differences when you consider your own baby. Your diet, where and how you live, your genetic makeup, hormonal changes—the list goes on—also contribute to your baby's health. While breastmilk is amazing, supplementing with formula or switching to formula if need be is not the end of the world.

Your Baby's Output

Your baby should have four to six wet diapers a day of about 6 tablespoons of urine. Her bowel movements will be less consistent after six weeks. Although she should have an average of one or more a day, don't be surprised if she skips a day and then presents you with a huge blowout. As she gets bigger, she may even go a week or more between poopy diapers. As long as she's gaining weight and not colicky, don't be alarmed. Breastmilk tends to create softer, runnier stools, and formula makes them firmer, but not hard.

Pumping

Pumping has likely found a place in your breastfeeding schedule. Whether it's a big morning pump to make your full breasts easier to latch on to, or a nightly pump so you can get a few more hours of sleep while your partner feeds the baby, it's a necessary part of breastfeeding. As your baby gets bigger and can go for longer stretches without you, you may want to venture out once in a while without her. While you may have settled into your favorite brand or style of pump, one thing that will continue to be challenging is where you do it.

There are hands-free portable pumps that allow you to hook yourself up and walk around. You can also engage with your baby in playtime while you pump to increase oxytocin. Hand pumps are great because you can use them anywhere. You may want to carry one around in your purse in case you need to pump while you're out or get delayed getting home to your electric one. Hand pumps are also helpful for clogged ducts, because you can change the angle to get to particular areas. There is a learning curve to these things. You may want to experiment with different pumping patterns, like using short bursts at first to stimulate your letdown and then switching to longer, slower pumps to get out more milk.

Getting the right-size flange is important. Choose one that fits all your nipple and part of your areola. The flange should feel comfortable, without friction, and allow for the most milk to come out without blocking the duct openings in your nipples. There are also elastic flanges made of polypropylene or silicone if the hard plastic ones are too difficult to use.

As time goes on, make sure you are cleaning your pump regularly. Also check the tubing for leaks or mold growths. If you rent a hospital-grade pump or any other shared pump, make sure to wipe it down well and often.

If you are returning to work, here are a few things to keep in mind. Although you have a legal right to pump at work, it's often hard to find a private place to do it. Depending on the kind of work you do, you may not have your own office, or you may have to travel to different locations. You may also not have control over your time, which makes scheduling three sessions a day challenging. I was in residency when I was pumping, so I had to lock myself in the call room and pray no one would come in. I also had a hard time scheduling breaks during surgeries, so I lived in constant fear of leaking if the cases went too long. Scope out places to pump beforehand. There are even websites that list locations you can use for pumping.

You will also need a fridge to store your milk, with an insulated container that is clearly marked. While you pump, look at pictures of your baby or think about her to encourage your letdown. It's also a good idea to keep some extra tops and nursing pads at work in case you leak. See Chapter 14 about returning to work.

Storing Breastmilk

If you are pumping milk, you will need to store it in the refrigerator or freezer. The cold can reduce the living cells in your milk, and freezing it can break down immunoglobulins. Even so, reheated breastmilk is still good for your baby.

After you pump, your milk can stay at room temperature for four to six hours, in the fridge for four days, or in the freezer for six to twelve months. If you don't use refrigerated milk right away, you can freeze it after four days of being in the fridge.

The easiest way to store pumped milk is with storage bags. They are clean and disposable, and don't take up a lot of room in the freezer or fridge. Just make sure they are made specifically for storing breastmilk. Even though they come with pre-printed markers for measuring how much milk they contain, they are notorious for being inaccurate. Double-check amounts by using a measuring cup or scale. If you prefer not to create waste, you can use clean food-grade jars or bottles. Recycled bottles may be made of plastic that contains BPA, so make sure they don't have a recycle number 7 on them. When you fill the bottle or bag, remember to leave extra room, because liquid expands when it cools.

When storing milk, make sure you label the bags or bottles with the date and time you pumped the milk. Use the older milk first. It's also better to store milk in one-time-use portions so you don't waste the extra. If you are not near a fridge or freezer, you can use an insulated bag with ice or ice packs to keep milk cool for up to twenty-four hours.

Reheating Breastmilk

When feeding refrigerated milk to your baby, you don't have to reheat it. Cold milk isn't dangerous for her. Some babies don't mind cold milk, depending on how hungry they are.

Most moms prefer to reheat milk regardless. The safest way to do so is by placing the bag or bottle in a container of hot liquid or under hot running water. Once the warmed milk is in the bottle, shake it to mix in the fatty parts and check to make sure it is not too hot. The right temperature is one you can't feel.

Microwaving breastmilk is tempting, but try not to fall for this quick fix. If you microwave breastmilk for more than five to ten seconds, you risk denaturing the immunoglobulins and rendering them useless. Theoretically, because microwaves heat unevenly, pockets of hot milk could burn your baby's mouth. Shaking or stirring the milk could prevent that, but you shouldn't be "cooking" your milk, so don't use a microwave. The same goes for pouring breastmilk into a pan and heating it over the stove. Bad idea, unless you want to make breastmilk pudding.

Frozen breastmilk takes a little longer to use. The safest way to thaw it is by putting it in the fridge overnight. But if all you have is frozen milk and you need it right away, warm it slowly by putting it in a pot of warm, not hot, water. This will take about ten to fifteen minutes, so it's not an immediate fix. Once you thaw frozen milk, you should use it within twenty-four hours. Once the crystals have thawed and it's no longer slushy, you should not refreeze milk.

If your baby doesn't finish a bottle of breastmilk, no matter how it was stored or even if it came right from you, you can keep it for up to two hours at room temperature. It's best not to try and salvage it by throwing it in the fridge, because it can have bacteria from your baby's mouth.

Using Bottles

If you are using bottles of stored milk or formula, you should consider the kind of nipple you're using. Yes, there are a ton of different nipple shapes and brands with promises of preventing colic or being more like your nipples. Your baby may have a preference for one style over another, but the truth is, none feel, or flow, like you.

When considering bottle nipples, understand that the "levels" are not medically or scientifically developed. They merely correlate to the number and size of holes in the nipples as follows. The age range is entirely made up by the manufacturers:

- *Level 1:* one hole—newborn to 3 months
- *Level 2:* two holes—3 to 6 months
- *Level 3:* three holes—6 to 9 months
- *Level 4:* four holes—9 to 12 months
- *Y-cut:* one large hole the shape of a *Y*—9 months and older

Moms are often told to use "low flow" nipples so their baby works harder to get the milk from a bottle, so it mimics the breast. This assumes two things: (1) Breastfeeding should be difficult, and (2) bottle nipples are anything like breasts. All nipples are made of silicone or rubber, not flesh. They are harder and more rigid than real nipples and don't conform to the inside of your baby's mouth like your breasts. Even the newer, fancier-shaped bottles with angled nipples and complicated venting don't replicate you. They also don't feel or smell like you.

Using bottles won't make your baby prefer them over you unless she has trouble transferring milk out of your breasts or you have a very low supply. I know this is a controversial statement, but so many babies have trouble gaping and latching deeply, it is a common problem for babies. Moms are told to avoid bottle nipples instead of addressing the underlying cause. Your baby is hardwired to prefer you over any other way to eat. But if she repeatedly tries to nurse without getting milk, she grows hungry and frustrated. When you follow it with a bottle, she will *learn* to prefer the bottle.

Positioning

As your baby gets bigger, you will need fewer props and pillows to nurse. Although some moms love the support that nursing pillows provide, once your baby has head control and starts moving on her own, the way you nurse changes as well.

Nursing in Public

As much as we believe nursing is wholesome and wonderful, it is still uncomfortable to nurse in public. A big reason is that Americans have a problem with naked female nipples. In 2014, the filmmaker Lina Esco made a documentary called *Free the Nipple,* which followed a group of women who took to the streets to raise awareness about the legal and cultural taboos of exposed female breasts. The film grew into a movement, still alive today, that includes demanding protection for breastfeeding moms.

This raises the question of why naked nipples are such a problem to begin with. Did you know that in the United States, Hawaii, New York, New Hampshire, Maine, Ohio, and Texas are the only states to legalize toplessness for men and women in public places? Thirty-seven states have laws that implicitly or explicitly state that any exposure of female nipples is considered a criminal offense for indecent exposure, and five of those states include breastfeeding. Only nine states, New York included, expressly differentiate breastfeeding mothers from public lewdness. Which leads me to wonder, how is pulling out your breast to feed your baby in public an infraction of *other* people's rights?

Although there is a difference between wanting to feed your baby and walking around topless in public for the hell of it, we may not be able to separate the two. From birth, we are socialized to believe that post-pubescent female nipples are taboo. They are covered up in magazines, allowed only in R-rated movies, and, when accidentally exposed on national television, cause more controversy than bloody war footage. They are even banned on social media.

But perhaps it is this very "hiding" of female nipples that makes them so exciting when you do catch a glimpse. Even though breastfeeding is natural, we are sensitized to believe that naked female breasts are primarily sexual. When someone heckles or stares at you breastfeeding your baby in public, I bet the emotion they are feeling is shame. They want you to stop so they don't have to deal with their own discomfort. But that's their problem. If they saw female nipples everywhere, maybe they would stop noticing or caring. Free the Nipple indeed. Feed your baby wherever you want to.

PART THREE

Failure to Feed: What Goes Wrong and What to Do About It

Pain, No Gain:
On Nipple and Breast Pain

The most common downside of breastfeeding is pain–pain with latching, pain during nursing, pain after nursing. But, for some reason, it is rarely taken seriously. Instead, you get mixed messages and generalizations that cause more confusion than clarification. In the same breath you are promised that nursing is supposed to feel good, you are also assured that breastfeeding pain is completely normal. Besides the obvious paradox, no one even explains what kind of pain they are talking about. All pain is put into one category, lumped together and brushed aside, effectively brainwashing moms into expecting it.

Pain may be common, but it's not normal. There are many varieties of breastfeeding pain, from mild and unavoidable to severe and potentially life-threatening. Pain can also be a powerful diagnostic tool, if you pay attention. It hurts because your body is trying to tell you something. Listen to it. If you break down the pain and examine it, the differences can help you figure out what's going wrong so you can look for ways to fix it.

Although pain can affect your mood, sleep, and energy level and make it nearly impossible to bond with your baby, it isn't just bad for you. It also means your baby is struggling in some very real way. Your pain can alert you that your baby isn't getting enough milk. It can also hint at why he has colic and cries all the time. If you ignore these clues, or just suffer like you're told to, you may miss the chance to correct the problem. As we know, breastfeeding is all about timing. Don't wait until it's too late.

For clarification, when someone tells you, "Pain is normal," what they really mean is a little pain for the first few days is expected. Breastfeeding is a learned skill, and although you and your baby are equipped with reflexes, you still have to sync up with each other to get it right. Engorgement as your breasts fill up–that can hurt. Their firm, more solid shape can make it harder for your baby to latch on–that hurts. Not latching your baby on deeply enough because you don't know how to hold all the parts together–that hurts too. That is the extent of expected breastfeeding pain. Anything other than that is not okay. I repeat, anything other than a little pain for the first few days means something is wrong, no matter what anyone tells you. Pain can happen, but it is not a necessary part of breastfeeding.

In this chapter, we will discuss pain in detail, along with the very real ramifications of ignoring it. We will differentiate between nipple and breast pain, discussing the underlying causes of both. We will also talk about the quantifiable measures of pain, why it persists, and the repercussions of ignored pain, like infections, plugged ducts, decreased supply, and a higher risk of postpartum depression.

"No pain, no gain" may be true for many parts of life, but it's not true for breastfeeding. Breastfeeding is supposed to be your reward for making a new human. You should be reveling in feel-good hormones that make nursing easier, not screaming in toe-curling agony every time your baby latches on. Don't defend your pain. Breastfeeding may take some work, but you don't have to be a martyr.

Now let's dive into how the shape of your nipples and breasts affects your breastfeeding experience.

Nipple Shape and Size

Regardless of their shape and size, nipples get blamed for breastfeeding woes almost as much as breasts do. Your nipples may be large and bulbous or round and taut, just like a bottle nipple. Some nipples are flat, others inverted. When your baby latches on right away, your nipples are lauded. When he can't, they are blamed. All this despite how differently they are all shaped.

Over the years, moms have told me hilarious stories about how they were told their "tiny" nipples are perfect for breastfeeding or their "flat" nipples are the reason their baby falls off the breast. If everything is going well, your nipples will get most of the credit. If not, you will be told they are too round, flat, big, small, sensitive, inverted—you name it. But here's the truth: Although your nipple shape can affect nursing, it is not nearly as important as you have been made to believe. Your nipples aren't *too* anything. They are perfect just the way they are.

Nipples are the part of your breasts that carry the openings of your milk ducts. They also happen to have the highest touch sensitivity of any other part of your breast. Keeping your nipples happy goes a long way toward keeping your whole milk supply going. When your baby is able to gape and latch normally, he can nurse from any nipple shape and it should feel good.

On another note, if you have nipple piercings, you may have trouble nursing. Horizontal piercings can cross your milk ducts, damaging them so milk can't come out. Removing the piercing is usually enough to correct the problem, but, on rare occasions, you may need surgery, depending on the damage.

FLAT AND INVERTED NIPPLES

About a third of moms have flat or inverted nipples, yet they are rarely the cause of nipple pain or a poor latch. Flat nipples are just that. They look and feel like the central part of the areola.

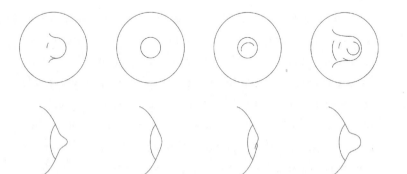

Figure 1 (in columns): Normal   *Figure 2: Flat*   *Figure 3: Inverted*   *Figure 4: Large*

While their shape may not create an obvious teat for your baby to latch on to, if your baby has a normal gape, he will be able to fit around your nipple and receive milk through it. Pressing or holding your breast in a sandwich shape and holding it there while nursing can help him stay latched.

Inverted nipples are different. Inversions happen when your nipple actually sticks to the tissue underneath, preventing it from protruding outward. Inverted nipples are usually something you are born with, but they can also happen from surgery, breast cancer, previous nursing, infections, or heavy breasts. One or both nipples can be affected.

You can tell the difference between flat and inverted nipples by pinching your areola an inch behind the nipple. If your nipple sticks out, it is flat. If not, it's inverted. Pumping or using breast shells can help draw your nipples out, or you can use the Hoffman Technique. This is done by placing your thumbs on each side of the base of your nipple then pushing your thumbs down and away from one another. This stretches your nipple and loosens the tissue underneath. You can do this exercise two to five times a day.

Sometimes inverted nipples can be more severely and permanently stuck to underlying tissue. In these cases, fibrosis and scarring can pull the milk ducts into the breast. If this happens, milk can't come out of your nipples. If you suspect this is a problem, see your OB/GYN for an evaluation. Surgery may be needed to stretch or lengthen the ducts. This is very rare.

Breast Shape and Size

Before breastfeeding, your breasts were probably pretty familiar to you. But once you start lactating, they take on a life of their own. Your breasts may grow to epic proportions or swell, then shrink down to tiny nubbins when you stop nursing. Some become pendular and amorphous, others hard and firm.

There is a wide range of breast shape and size, even on the same mom. Your two breasts may grow in opposite ways, one filling to a gentle B cup while the other grows down to your belly button. But don't let their size fool you. Even though you may call your smaller breast the *bad* one, it may actually produce more milk than the larger one. In case you hadn't noticed, your breasts are not twins. They are sisters. And, when you breastfeed, they may feel like they are from another planet.

Despite what you may have been told, your breast size and shape is not reason your baby can't latch on. Even though your breasts get blamed for breastfeeding failure almost as much as your nipples, as long as your baby is able to gape normally, he will be able to latch on to any breast shape. If he can't gape, he won't be able to latch on to any breast. The one exception is during the first few days of engorgement, when most breasts are hard and full. Pumping off a little milk to soften your breasts can make latching easier.

Your breast shape and size also does not determine whether you will be able to breastfeed, with two exceptions: if you've had breast surgery to remove a significant amount of breast tissue or if you were born with *hypoplastic breasts,* which have very little glandular tissue. In both cases, you may struggle with supply. There are also medical and hormonal reasons for low supply. Issues with supply will be discussed in Chapter 11.

Nipple Pain

It is important to distinguish between *nipple* and *breast* pain. We will first talk about nipple pain, although they often happen together.

Nipple pain is caused primarily by *friction*. Friction happens when you rub your sensitive nipples over and over again. It's the same reason a man's nipples hurt when he goes for a run with a loose-fitting T-shirt. It is also why pumping hurts if you don't have a flange that fits well. Your poor nipple moves in and out of a flange that's too big or gets trapped in one that's too small.

Friction happens when your baby is not latched on to your breast deeply enough. When he is latched well, his mouth forms a seal over your areola, and your nipple stays tucked deep in his throat, where nothing is touching it. If he can't gape, your nipple sits more forward in his mouth, and his sucking movements rub right on your nipples instead of your areola or breast. It's that friction that does all the damage. Rawness, bleeding, scabbing, and even yeast infections are all a result of friction. Over the years I've seen nipples slaughtered by friction. There is no end to the suffering that moms will endure for their babies. The saddest part is that it isn't worth it.

Nipple pain is always bad and mostly stems from a shallow latch. You have to address the underlying problem, but you can take a break to let your nipples heal in the short term. You can try different creams, ointments, and salves like glycerine gel, lanolin, coconut oil, peppermint gel, and expressed breastmilk. You may be tempted to slap on a nipple shield to dull the pain. You can treat the infections caused by nipple friction and damage (see below), but none of these treatments will stop friction unless you address the underlying problem. And the most common reason for friction is your baby's *restricted gape* (see Chapter 10).

Over time, nursing with a shallow latch may become less painful, but it's not because your baby's latch gets better. The damage from repeated friction can cause a loss of sensation and scarring—that toughening-up process everyone talks about. While there are some moms who can nurse through pain, sometimes for years, it's pretty rare. Even if they can tolerate the torture, they will eventually lose their supply if they don't pump. Nipple pain is a sign that your breasts aren't getting emptied fully. Even if the pain subsides and the cracks heal, you still have to address the underlying cause of friction. Otherwise, you may run into trouble with your supply when you least expect it. See Chapter 13 for options.

NIPPLE INFECTION

Nipple infections are a common cause of pain, and they are usually superficial. They can be viral (*Herpes simplex*), bacterial, fungal, or mixed. Usually, nipple infections follow nipple damage because broken skin can be a source of infection. Infections rarely happen without prolonged friction, so look for an underlying cause. Yeast infections are most common and tend to be less painful than bacterial infections.

Topical creams, like Neosporin and Monistat, can cure nipple infections. Lanolin or coconut oil alone usually isn't enough. If you like home remedies, a salve made of white vinegar and baking soda placed on your nipples twice a day can heal nearly any infection. Use just enough vinegar to make a paste, let it air-dry, and wipe it off before feeding your baby or pumping. It may sting at first, but after a few days your symptoms should go away.

RAYNAUD'S PHENOMENON

Around 20 percent of women of childbearing age have something called Raynaud's phenomenon.[1] Raynaud's is caused by tiny arteries spasming in extremities like fingers, toes, and nipples. Because of the lack of blood flow, people with Raynaud's can develop painful stinging when exposed to cold or pressure. When the arteries spasm, extremities can turn white and then red or blue from lack of oxygen.

Diagnosing Raynaud's on your painful nipples can be tricky because you have to first distinguish between it and friction from a bad latch. If you have Raynaud's, you usually develop symptoms before pregnancy and breastfeeding. Symptoms happen with cold alone, and not just with pressure. When you are having spasms, your extremities go through two or three color changes, not just blanching from being compressed. Sometimes Raynaud's is misdiagnosed as a fungal infection, and you figure out it's Raynaud's only because the medication doesn't help. To make it more confusing, Raynaud's can cause nipple pain even when your baby is latched on correctly. The good news is that it's rare. Your doctor can prescribe a medication called nifedipine, but it is usually offered only after everything else has been ruled out.

Breast Pain

Breast and nipple pain often go hand in hand, which makes sense. If your baby can't latch on deeply because of a restricted gape, you will likely have nipple pain from friction, but you will also have backup in milk flow out of your breast. That backup can lead to engorgement, plugged ducts, and, when combined with nipple damage, mastitis. But you can develop these problems even without nipple pain and a shallow latch. Breast pain without nipple pain is mostly related to backup in milk and blood flow. Let's discuss each in detail.

ENGORGEMENT

You may wake up one morning, early on, with terrible breast pain. Your breasts may be hard and red and warm all over. You may even have a low-grade fever. Because they're so huge, your nipples may look flatter, making it harder for your baby to latch on. This is engorgement. It is both a blessing and a curse.

Engorgement is most common during the first three to seven days of nursing, when the blood flow to your breasts increases and you start making transitional milk. Engorgement is also common during the first few weeks, when milk gets backed up in your breasts as you are trying to sync up your supply with your baby's needs. Maybe you were out and couldn't find a place to pump, or you make a lot of milk, but your baby isn't fully draining your breasts. If you don't empty your breasts or if they fill too quickly, blood can also back up in your veins—something called *venous congestion.* This over-stretching of your breasts not only hurts, but also makes it harder to drain them. The increased blood in your breasts makes them so taut, the milk ducts get compressed so it's harder for the milk to come out.

In one way, engorgement is a good sign because it means your milk is coming in. On the other, you have to do some-thing about it or you could develop plugged ducts or an infec-tion, such as mastitis. As with every other part of the body that makes fluid (think saliva glands and bladders), it comes down to plumbing. If the fluid can't come out, it backs up and causes even more problems.

The best way to deal with engorgement is to make sure you empty your breasts every two to three hours. You can try warm compresses to get the milk flowing and cold compresses to bring the swelling down. You can even pump out a little before nursing to make it easier for your baby to latch on and form a seal. The key is to keep your breasts empty as often as possible, so you keep your supply going and avoid a breast infection. Remember all that stuff about prolactin, FIL, and oxytocin? It is important to keep the supply and demand going to get through the engorgement period with minimal pain and constant flow.

PLUGGED DUCTS

As we know, milk is made deep in your breasts, in little sacs called alveoli. Once they fill, the milk drains through tubes, called ducts. And if the ducts don't drain, the fluid backs up. If the fluid backs up, you may feel hard cords in your breast that are tender to the touch. These hard cords are called *plugged ducts,* even though the term is a misnomer. The hard lumps you feel deep in your breasts when you can't empty them are actually full alveoli, so the ducts can't drain the milk.

Plugged ducts are different from engorgement. They usually happen later, when engorgement has passed. One or more ducts can be blocked, but it usually doesn't involve your whole breast. They can happen if your baby isn't transferring milk efficiently. They can also happen if you make a lot more milk than your baby needs and you aren't pumping enough. Just like engorgement, plugged ducts can lead to infection and a decrease in supply, over time, if they aren't addressed.

Dealing with plugged ducts can be tricky. Massaging your breast before, during, and after you pump or nurse is helpful. So is using a warm compress, like a microwaved wet towel, or soaking your breasts in an Epsom salt bath. Some lactation consultants recommend sunflower lecithin as an oral supplement to resolve plugged ducts. No one knows exactly why this works, but it could be that lecithin helps the fatty part of your milk stay suspended in the sugary part. Regardless of the method you use, it must always be followed by emptying your breasts. You can use your baby or pump.

The dangling nursing position helps (see Chapter 7). Hand pumps may be most helpful, because you can target the plugged ducts directly.

MASTITIS

Mastitis is fancy word for infected breast. If it sadly happens to you, it doesn't feel fancy at all. It feels miserable. It can come on suddenly and make you develop a high fever, sudden breast pain, body aches, and chills. Your breasts will be red, swollen, and warm to the touch. They will also be very, very painful. Mastitis is no joke and should never be ignored.

As dramatic as mastitis sounds, it is also surprisingly common. Up to a third of moms develop it. It is usually caused by the one-two punch of damaged nipples and backed-up milk flow. The damage to your nipples allows bacteria commonly found on your skin, called *Staphylococcus aureus,* to enter the bloodstream around your breasts. Pools of nutrient-rich milk in your breasts make a delicious food supply, very quickly growing millions of bacteria. Combine that with the increase in blood flow into and out of your lactating breasts, and you can see how easily more severe infections, like *sepsis,* a blood infection, or a breast abscess can develop.

Mastitis can happen even without nipple damage from prolonged engorgement or plugged ducts. If your baby can't transfer your milk out completely or if you make more than your baby needs, milk backs up. Like any other part of your body, when fluid sits for too long, it can get infected. If you have a big supply, you are more prone to mastitis, engorgement, and plugged ducts even if your baby seems to be transferring milk effectively.

Symptoms of mastitis can spread so quickly; you can get sick within a few hours. If you think you have it, seek medical care immediately. Treatment is usually ten to fourteen days of antibiotics, and your doctor may or may not do a milk culture. If you develop a breast abscess, you will need surgical drainage along with antibiotics. In more serious cases or if you develop sepsis, you may need to be hospitalized for intravenous antibiotics.

Another downside to mastitis is that even one bout of it can greatly reduce your supply. If it happens over and over again, you risk losing more supply each time. It isn't normal to have recurrent mastitis, so if it keeps happening, feel around your breasts for masses or cysts, as they can block the flow of milk out of your ducts.

As with plugged ducts and engorgement, the key to preventing mastitis is consistent removal of milk from your breasts. It's okay to keep nursing as long as the antibiotics you are given are safe for your baby. But keep in mind that mastitis often happens when your baby doesn't have a deep latch. If you have nipple pain with nursing and frequent bouts of plugged ducts, it may be better to focus on pumping and emptying while you look into underlying problems related to your baby's latching and transfer. One mom I treated had frequent bouts of mastitis, and no matter how much she pumped or took antibiotics, it kept coming back. When we addressed her baby's shallow latch and got him nursing effectively, her mastitis completely resolved.

Postpartum Depression

Pain can affect much more than breastfeeding. In addition to the obvious physical trauma, it can cause emotional trauma as well. Of course, anyone who is subjected to repeated pain gets depressed and angry. But new moms have it even worse. Even beyond the stress of not sleeping and caring for and feeding a new baby, postpartum pain can cause very real *hormonal* changes. And these hormones can affect the physiology and the way your brain functions, even after you stop nursing.

To understand why, let's think back to our discussion about oxytocin. In addition to causing your letdown, oxytocin also induces a state of bliss and calm in you and promotes bonding with your baby. We tend to think of oxytocin being released only when you nurse. But just thinking about your baby, smelling him, touching him, seeing him, or even hearing his cry also stimulates its release. Feeling good makes your brain release even more oxytocin. And the same goes for your baby. It's this reciprocal hormonal release that creates bonding, a physiologic connection between the two of you. When considering the power of oxytocin, one study showed that complete strangers behaved more kindly and lovingly toward one another after hugging. Imagine the power of repeated, reinforced oxytocin between you and your baby. You would literally do anything to show your love.

Now imagine what would happen if you turned this whole system on its head. What would happen if, instead of feeling bliss and calm, you felt pain when you latched your baby on? How would that pain affect your hormones? First off, you wouldn't release oxytocin. Your breasts would hold on to your milk, causing engorgement or plugged ducts. You wouldn't be filled with a rush of love toward your baby; instead, you would learn to associate pain with him. That association would make you feel guilty, so you would try to overcome it by putting up with even more pain to prove you love him.

No matter how much you soldier on, your baby would develop negative associations with nursing from you. Without oxytocin, your letdown would be subdued, and your baby would have to work harder to get milk. If it hurts you, he probably isn't very efficient to begin with, so making him nurse without the benefit of a letdown only makes nursing harder for him. He would soon learn that you, your smell, your breasts, won't give him what he needs. His brain would produce less oxytocin when he goes to your breast.

Your physical pain also makes your body release *cortisol,* a hormone produced in your adrenal glands. It is released in times of stress and causes you to feel anxiety, fear, and panic. If you have high enough levels of cortisol in your bloodstream, it can even delay your milk production, reinforcing those negative associations. Over time, you start to feel sad because your brain doesn't release as much *dopamine,* a hormone that makes you feel happy and excited. Dopamine is also stimulated by oxytocin release, and the two hormones reinforce each other. With all that cortisol and so little oxytocin and dopamine, before you know it, you could develop *postpartum depression (PPD).* And there isn't anything you can think or believe or "get over" to help you through it.

PPD is a serious mental health condition that occurs in

nearly one-fifth of moms who have recently given birth. Its symptoms are a persistent low mood, feelings of worthlessness, sadness, hopelessness, panic attacks, and difficulty bonding with your baby. It usually starts within the first six weeks to six months after you have your baby. It's different than "baby blues," which happen in 80 percent of moms who get similar symptoms within the first few days of giving birth. The difference between the two is that baby blues go away after ten days, and PPD continues on.

By the time a new mom has suffered even a week of painful nursing, she is at increased risk of developing PPD. This is because the pain creates a physiologic hormonal depression and feelings of hopelessness. With too much cortisol and too little oxytocin, bonding is affected as well, creating even more shame. One study showed that when moms stopped breast-feeding because of pain, they were more likely to develop PPD.[2] That higher risk of PPD lasted for up to six months after they stopped nursing. Not all PPD is a consequence of pain from breastfeeding, but I am convinced that pain causes far more PPD than we even consider.

When you have PPD, it's hard to ask for help because you don't even realize what is happening. Your mood depends on your hormones. By the way, this is true of everyone, not just perinatal women. We are *all* controlled by our hormones. It's hard to tell the difference between normal new mother exhaustion and PPD, especially when it first happens. Thankfully, pediatricians and obstetricians are getting better at diagnosing it. If symptoms are severe enough, please do seek help; you may need medication or hospitalization. You don't have to continue to suffer alone. If you do develop PPD, make sure you conduct a thorough evaluation of your breastfeeding experience. The root of the problem may actually be hidden in there and totally fixable.

Dysphoric Milk Ejection Reflex (D-MER)

A relatively new condition that is coming to light is something called *dysphoric milk ejection reflex,* or *D-MER.* D-MER is when a breastfeeding mom has a surge of negative emotions about thirty to ninety seconds before her letdown. This can happen with breastfeeding or pumping. By the time her milk is released, her bad feelings go away, but they come back just before every other letdown.

The negative emotions can be mild, like a sigh or hollow feeling in your stomach. But they can also be worse, ranging from sadness and nervousness to dread and hopelessness, and sometimes even suicidality. Something just very suddenly feels very wrong. And just like that, after your letdown, all those feelings disappear. For some moms, D-MER symptoms get better after three months, but for others they continue the whole time they breastfeed.

Very little research has been done on D-MER, but the current theory is that it is a physiologic problem caused by dysfunction of the hormone dopamine. When considering the symptoms, however, *serotonin* is a more likely culprit. Serotonin is a hormone that makes you feel calm when you have anxiety. Interestingly, the way serotonin acts in your brain changes with pregnancy and postpartum.[3] The important point is that D-MER is not psychological. Just like PPD, you can't stop these feelings, because they are controlled by your hormones.

Although PPD and D-MER are different conditions, they sometimes overlap and respond to different treatments. Treatment for D-MER is mostly through awareness and understanding of what is happening when cases are mild or moderate. Eating or doing something distracting can help you get through the surge of symptoms. Avoiding stress and getting enough sleep (good luck with that) can also make symptoms less awful. Severe cases may require herbal or medical treatment, but D-MER is generally not a huge deterrent to breastfeeding. Like I said, moms will go through almost anything for their babies.

It's Not You, It's the Baby:
Gape Restriction and Tongue Tie

Now that you know the mechanics of breastfeeding, I'm sure we can agree that it's a complicated process. But when all is well, it should work like a well-oiled machine. Your baby should easily empty your breasts and get lots of milk, and it should feel good for both of you.

Except when it doesn't.

In truth, only half of moms are able to nurse right off the bat. The other half struggle. And by struggle, I mean anything from irritating pain to impossible hell. It's easy to get lost in techniques and timing and pumping regimens and nursing positions. When you run into trouble, it's also easy to assume it's your fault. Even if you don't blame yourself, everyone else will. You will be told you're too stressed, or your breasts are too soft/large/small/round/flat, or you aren't holding your baby correctly or getting her to latch deeply. No matter the excuse, you will get the credit for failure.

Here's a secret: Most of the time, it's not you. It's your baby.

As I've mentioned several times (it's important!), the most

common culprit in your breastfeeding struggle is your baby's inability to gape. Because gape is the first step in latching, if it fails, so does everything that comes after it. Restricted gape is the single greatest cause for failed breastfeeding, yet it's never fully explained. Moms are just told to get their baby to open wide. When she doesn't, moms are told to move on to the latch and ignore that step one didn't even happen.

With a restricted gape, your baby may not be able to open her mouth much at all. Her mouth may even look small. Even if she can open wide, she won't be able to stay that way, so she will slide down to your nipple where you can *feel* the problem. It hurts, it's frustrating, and you nurse forever but your baby will still be hungry. To make matters worse, no one can see the problem, because you can't see a latch from the outside. Only you can feel it.

And remember, if your baby doesn't gape when she's born, it's not because she won't. It's because she can't. Massaging her mouth with exercises won't fix it. Trying to pull her mouth open doesn't help either, because gape restriction is an anatomic problem. When your baby is born, she can either gape or she can't. If she can't gape, she will never be able to nurse normally without an intervention. On the other hand, if you decide not to nurse, gape restriction doesn't matter.

In this chapter we will talk about gape restriction in detail and how your baby's anatomy causes it. We will also talk about tongue tie, the misuse of the terms *posterior tongue tie* and *lip tie* and how they were coined, along with options for managing gape restriction. I will discuss the ethics of intervention, with a warning about the growing number of dentists and doctors who dabble in procedures with little to no formal training, regulatory oversight, or understanding of the anatomy.

Anatomy That Causes Gape Restriction

Although nursing is natural, nature is messy. So it goes with your baby's gape. Some babies cannot gape wide enough to unhinge their jaw when they are born. How, you may ask, have we been able to survive as a species this way? If babies can't nurse from their own mom, won't they starve? (The answer is no. There are a lot of ways to feed a baby.)

Poor fit is typical of nature. Take childbirth, for example. Not every baby can fit through her mom's birth canal without help. That's why we need C-sections and forceps. Why should breastfeeding be any different? Sometimes things fit perfectly. Sometimes they don't. It all boils down to anatomy.

The most common cause for gape restriction is how your baby's head is shaped and how the roof of her mouth, tongue, and jaw are positioned. When your baby is developing, her head shape is determined by the way she sits in your womb. If she is able to move around a lot, her head will be rounder. If she can't, her soft skull bones will be molded by your sturdier bony parts. For example, if she is breech for the last trimester, the part of her head that sits under your rib will be compressed when she comes out. Similarly, if she goes head down early in the third trimester, her head will be molded by the shape of the inside of your pelvic girdle and look oblong or cone-shaped when she is born.

Any womb position where your baby stays tucked in one place will shift the axis of her head and affect all the structures on the inside. Specifically, with her head tucked, her jaw position will move back and up a little more than usual. This is called *retrognathia*. Her palate, or roof of her mouth, will also change from the typical horizontal shape to a more vertical, arched shape. Her tongue, however, will stay in the same position. But because her tongue is connected to the floor of her mouth, the shift in her jaw position will prevent her tongue from being able to move normally. The subtle shift in the axis of your baby's head makes her tongue, jaw, and palate move together instead of independently.

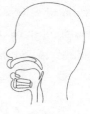

Figure 1: Normal,
open mouth

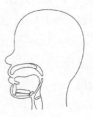

Figure 2: Normal,
closed mouth

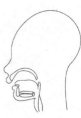

Figure 3: High palate,
set-back jaw, open mouth

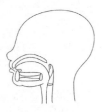

Figure 4: High palate,
set-back jaw, closed mouth

If this is too complicated to understand, imagine one of those Transformer toys. Because of the way the parts are connected, you have to move each piece in a particular order to *transform* the toy from one shape to another. Now imagine melting or pressing the toy into a different shape and then trying to move the pieces around. It won't work.

The same goes for your baby's anatomy. If the axis of your baby's head is more oblong, she won't be able to unhinge her jaw, because the parts are attached differently. Dropping her jaw will actually pull her tongue down, away from her palate, so she won't be able to compress your breast. Pulling her tongue up to her palate will pull her jaw along with it, closing her mouth instead of keeping it open. Unhinging her jaw will be impossible. Instead, to open her mouth, she will have to hinge at her jaw and hold it there. Hinging takes a lot of effort. (Think about how hard it is to keep your mouth open at the dentist). After a while, her latch will slip down to your nipple—and ouch!

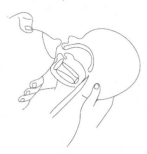

Figure 1: Restricted gape

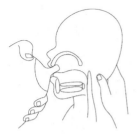

Figure 2: Shallow latch on the nipple

Without being able to unhinge her jaw, your baby will have a small gape. A small gape always results in a shallow latch. If your baby can't open her mouth wide enough, your nipple can't lock into position at the back of her throat. Her palate, which will be more arched, won't fill with enough breast to stimulate a normal suck reflex. Every time she sucks, she will take down air, leading to gas and colic. Sometimes she won't be able to suck at all. She will have a really hard time transferring milk on her own and will have to rely on your letdown. It's exhausting and frustrating, because she can smell the milk but she can't get it out.

Something else happens when your baby can't gape normally. If she tries and fails to nurse repeatedly, she will eventually lose her gape reflex. She will fall asleep at the breast, or stop opening her mouth once she gets there. Once she stops nursing, you will be forced to feed her from a bottle or other source. When she sees that she can get food another way, she will learn to purse her lips to pull in the bottle nipple instead of opening wide. Some babies adapt quickly, in a matter of days. In others it can take weeks. This is one form of *nipple confusion* and will be discussed in Chapter 12.

If you think your baby has gape restriction, you are probably right. It's easy for you to diagnose because you can see it every time you try to latch her on. You can also feel it because it is almost always painful. In fact, you will be able to diagnose gape restriction better than anyone else. Most lactation consultants and doctors ignore it completely, offering impossible advice instead of examining your baby's anatomy. They will tell you to hold your baby's mouth open or compress your breast into a panini and try to shove it in her mouth. But these things won't work. You need to first address the underlying anatomic problem before moving forward.

If your baby can't gape, the problem can be corrected. If you don't want to do an frenulectomy, there are other options, depending on your supply. Gape restriction matters only in the first year of life, for breastfeeding and sometimes for bottle-feeding. Once you are past the nursing and bottle phase, none of it matters. Her high palate and set-back jaw will correct themselves as she grows into her second year.

Tongue Tie

I'm sure everyone has heard the term *tongue tie* by now. It's literally on the tips of everyone's tongues, shouldering the blame for every breastfeeding frustration imaginable. Unfortunately, tongue tie is also terribly misunderstood and overdiagnosed. As an ear, nose, and throat doctor, I have been diagnosing and treating tongue tie in babies, children, and adults for nearly two decades. But before we discuss the pros and cons of treating it, we have to be clear on what tongue tie actually means.

When your baby is developing in your womb, her tongue starts out as two parts, then fuses down the middle into one structure. When that fusion happens, there is extra tissue that forms underneath her tongue to separate it from the floor of her mouth. That tissue is called a *frenulum*. Some frenulum is normal, but most of it is supposed to dissolve away, allowing her tongue to move freely. When that extra tissue doesn't dissolve, it holds her tongue down, preventing it from lifting up, moving back, and moving forward. That *extra* frenulum is called *tongue tie*. It happens in 4 to 10 percent of the general population and is thought to be genetic. If your baby has tongue tie, you will see a stringy thing under her tongue when she cries or opens her mouth. Although it looks stringy, tongue tie is really a three-dimensional piece of connective tissue that tents forward when she lifts up her tongue. Technically, a tongue is considered tied when 75 percent of that extra tissue doesn't dissolve. The tip of her tongue may also be heart-shaped from the frenulum tethering it in the middle. Tongue tie is kind of like being born with your shoelaces tied: You can walk, but it takes a lot of effort. Everyone has a frenulum, but not everyone has tongue tie.

Contrary to popular opinion, tongue tie never stretches out on its own. It also prevents your baby's tongue from developing normally. This can cause other, more permanent changes in her tongue and mouth. The tongue is a muscle, so its shape is determined by the way it moves. If you don't release tongue tie right away, your baby will have a smaller, less muscular tongue. She will also have a harder time licking things, moving food to the back of her throat, cleaning her teeth with her tongue, and lifting her tongue. It will affect her speech, making it harder to articulate certain sounds. Because her tongue can't lift to compress the roof of her mouth, her already arched palate will remain high and arched, leading to smaller nasal volume. Some adults with untreated tongue tie also have crowded lower teeth, jaw problems, and snoring.

There has been a lot of research and discussion about how tongue tie affects breastfeeding.[1] If tongue tie is severe enough, it can cause gape restriction and all the symptoms that go along with it. However, not all babies with tongue tie have trouble nursing. It depends on how they fit onto their mom's breasts and the strength of her milk flow. Even so, most moms have improvement in breastfeeding when their baby's tongue tie is released, even if they thought things were fine.

For all these reasons, it is important to release a tongue tie as soon and completely as possible. In babies less than a year old, this can be done as a simple office procedure and doesn't require anesthesia. The sooner you release a tongue tie, the less chance it will grow back. No matter how or when it's done, there is always regrowth to a certain degree, so the incision site should be stretched after it's released. If you wait until your baby is a toddler to release a tongue tie, she will need anesthesia if you take her to an ear, nose, and throat doctor. Her recovery will be more painful and take longer, and the tongue tie will have a greater chance of growing back. She may also need speech therapy to strengthen her tongue. Regrowth in adults can happen up to 85 percent of the time.

Patient Perspective

Jack was two weeks old when his mom brought him in to see me. He had been struggling to latch, opening his mouth and shaking his head back and forth over her nipples before settling in to nurse. When he was able to latch on, his mom nearly screamed from the pain for the first few minutes. Over time her pain lessened, but her nipples had become damaged, with bleeding and broken skin. Her supply seemed okay, though, and she was able to pump two to three ounces between feeds. Jack was gaining weight, so she had assumed he was doing fine and that the pain was just her problem. He had some gas and reflux, but was otherwise okay, and she felt like she was being selfish for bringing him in. Her pediatrician noticed he had tongue tie, so he referred her to see me.

On exam, he had a visible tongue tie and normally arched palate. After undergoing release of his tongue frenulum, he was able to latch on with a much wider gape. Mom still had some residual pain, but she could feel that he was latched on more deeply.

Posterior Tongue Tie and Lip Tie

While there is consensus that tongue tie causes problems nursing, there are many more babies who struggle to nurse and don't have tongue tie. These babies are being diagnosed with *posterior tongue tie* and *lip tie*. As I will explain, these terms are more of a misunderstanding of cause and effect than real diagnoses.

As early as the 1400s, midwives have been releasing tied tongues with sharp fingernails. In the 1970s, doctors started releasing them as well. Sadly, there was no consistency in treatment protocols, so the results had mixed success and were ultimately abandoned. In the early 2000s, tongue tie was rediscovered as a cause for breastfeeding difficulty, thanks to a small number of us who took interest and had success in treating them. By 2009, releasing tongue ties to help breastfeeding became popular again. But as we treated more babies, it was clear that there were many more struggling babies who didn't have tongue tie than those who did.

In an effort to figure out the paradox, Dr. Elizabeth Coryllos, a pediatric surgeon from Long Island, created a classification system.[2] But instead of differentiating tongue tie from a normal frenulum, she instead called *all* frenula tongue tie, and typed them based on what they looked like. If the baby had a visible tongue tie, it was called Type 1 or Type 2. If the frenulum was not visible, it was called Type 3 or 4, or posterior tongue tie. While this was a first step in understanding how tongue tie affects breastfeeding, she sadly passed away before she could clarify her case. In the many years since it was written, her method of classifying oral tethering into types of tongue tie has plagued the diagnosis of breastfeeding issues and created much debate and confusion.

The term *posterior tongue tie* is problematic for many reasons. Posterior tongue tie is not an anatomic structure. When you look in your baby's mouth, there is nothing to see, because posterior tongue tie just means the baby can't nurse, and there is *no* tongue tie. Some practitioners try to explain how the frenulum is thick and tethered in these babies, but the truth is, without knowing a baby's history, no one can diagnose posterior tongue tie by simply looking into a baby's mouth. Using "tongue tie" in the description is also misleading because these babies don't develop issues with speech or tongue movement. Furthermore, if you release a supposed posteriorly tied frenulum alone, it doesn't help breastfeeding.

Pediatricians rightly refute the existence of posterior tongue tie. Unfortunately, they don't have a better answer for breastfeeding problems. If a baby struggles to nurse, they usually recommend formula or pumping or refer you to a lactation consultant who then diagnoses posterior tongue tie. Many moms just go along with this confusing diagnosis because they want help. There is obviously a reason their baby can't nurse, but this is the wrong way to look at it.

What about the term *lip tie*? Is that also hogwash? Yes and no. A lip frenulum is present in *every* newborn. It is meant to hold a space between her baby teeth so there is room for her permanent teeth to come in. A lip frenulum alone does not predict whether a baby will have trouble nursing. While the diagnosis of lip tie exists, it is just a cosmetic deformity caused by a thick upper lip frenulum resulting in a gap between the front two teeth. Pediatric dentists recommend waiting until a child is nine years or older before deciding if it needs to be cut. If you don't cut a lip tie, it causes only a cosmetic problem. It won't affect speech or anything else. You can't predict or diagnose a lip tie in a newborn, because *every* baby has a lip frenulum. You have to wait until she is older to see if it will cause a gap. As with to posterior tongue tie, if you cut only the lip frenulum when a baby is having trouble nursing, her nursing won't improve.

Which brings us back to the question, What is causing all these nursing problems in babies who don't have tongue tie? You already know the answer. It's gape restriction. If someone diagnoses your baby with posterior tongue tie or lip tie–there are even cheek ties now–what they are really trying to say is that they don't know why you are struggling but they can't see a tongue tie. The real diagnosis is that your baby can't open her mouth wide enough. When she can't gape to unhinge her jaw, she instead hinges at her jaw. This causes a shallow latch. Her set-back jaw–not the frenulum–restricts her tongue movement and prevents her tongue from lifting up to reach her high, arched palate. Her upper lip curls under because of her high palate and the position of her jaw relative to her midface. She may also develop an upper-lip blister from friction.

The Notion of Fit

Which brings us back to the notion of fit. Unlike the use of wet nurses of the past, today's moms want to breastfeed their babies on their own breasts. Combined with the pressure to get everyone breastfeeding, it's no wonder so many moms need help. Moms have always had trouble breastfeeding. But they have also been resourceful, figuring out other ways to feed their babies, even if it means giving them animal milk. In terms of nursing, if your baby can't gape, she will not be able to latch on normally to any breast. Conversely, if your baby has a wide, normal gape, she will be able to latch on to any breast or nipple shape.

I think of tongue tie and gape restriction as two distinct but overlapping issues. They make a good Venn diagram.

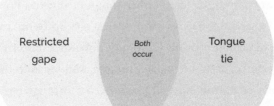

If your baby has tongue tie, it must be released as soon as possible. Sometimes clipping an obvious tongue tie improves the fit, and sometimes it doesn't. If it doesn't, your baby probably also has a high, arched palate and set-back jaw. It's important to treat both if you want to nurse. There are babies who have gape restriction without tongue tie, which is treated in a similar manner. Whether it's from tongue tie or gape restriction or both, your baby has to fit on to your breasts to be able to nurse.

MANAGING GAPE RESTRICTION

Now we finally get to the reason for all the confusion. It lies in the fact that the treatment for gape restriction is confused with its cause. Simply put, when your baby has gape restriction, even though the lip and tongue frenula aren't the problem, releasing both of them at the same time is the solution. The frenula are normal connective tissue, but because they serve no other purpose, cutting them when your baby has those anatomic shifts we talked about gets around the anatomy. Cutting the lower frenulum releases her tongue from the floor of the mouth and retrognathic jaw. Cutting the lip frenulum allows her lip to curl up instead of pulling down her hard palate. Releasing both allows her palate, tongue, and jaw to move freely. Freedom of movement will allow her to unhinge her jaw and gape. This works only if you release both frenula at the same time. If you release only one, there won't be improvement.[3]

I'll admit that understanding how this works is not intuitive. When I first started doing these procedures, I was shocked when I "fixed" the problem by cutting both frenula. I didn't even understand the problem fully at first. It took me another four years of research to figure out why these procedures worked and which problem they were fixing. By finding the solution, I was able to trace it back to the cause. Releasing the lip and tongue frenula allowed these babies to gape without restriction.

The timing of when to release frenula is debatable. I'm a fan of doing it as soon as you notice the problem for all the reasons we've already discussed. But because you need time to see how you and your baby fit, it makes sense to spend a week figuring it out first. Sometimes your baby won't fit because you're engorged. When your hard, swollen breasts get softer, her latch will improve. But if it's been a week and you are still struggling, she probably has gape restriction. You will have to decide whether you want to go for a procedure. Like I've said before, waiting for the pain to get better or her latch to improve is not the answer. You may not want a procedure, but the problem will remain.

Patient Perspective

Jaheem was a four-week-old baby who was not able to breastfeed well. His mom had a long labor, and he was ultimately born by C-section. She had to take steroids during her pregnancy for an underlying autoimmune problem, and thus had a hard time recuperating from the delivery. When she tried to nurse, her baby would get "violent" and wanted to eat frequently. When he tried to nurse, he could get only onto the nipple, and it was very painful for mom. He would nurse for a long time and still be hungry afterward. When mom pumped, she made thirty to forty milliliters in total, but she pumped only once a day.

On exam, Jaheem had a thick visible tongue tie and a high palate and set-back jaw. After undergoing upper and lower frenulectomies, he was able to gape more widely. Mom was able to nurse in the office without pain, but the baby became upset because she had little milk. Mom was advised to take supplements to boost her supply, and nurse for five to ten minutes on each side using a supplementary nursing system to entice the baby to continue nursing, followed by pumping for five minutes on each side.

The cutting of a frenulum is called *frenulectomy.* It should be performed in a controlled setting with a lot of light, using sterile instruments. Only the superficial tissue under the tongue and under the upper lip should be cut, never the underlying muscle. Cutting the tongue muscle causes terrible pain and a lot of bleeding. If the cut is too deep, the bleeding parts have to be burned or *cauterized,* which causes even more pain and makes recovery take longer. There will also be more scarring and regrowth. If your baby is less than a year old, frenulectomies can be done in an office setting, with topical numbing or no numbing at all. General anesthesia is never necessary, especially if it's done before your baby is a year old, and you can nurse right away afterward.

There are two ways to perform frenulectomies: using a laser or using sterile scissors. I have always used scissors, so I am biased toward them. They are very precise, and there is very little tissue damage. It is also easy for mom to hold the baby in her arms because the snips take less than five seconds. If done correctly, there is minimal bleeding, and the baby can nurse right away. Cauterizing is rarely needed because getting the baby breastfeeding stops the bleeding. Breastfeeding your baby is also soothing, and I can check that the procedure worked right away. There are many doctors who do frenulectomies and then cauterize the tissue, which causes more pain and scarring. As long as it's done in the right surgical plane and the baby latches on right away, there is rarely a reason for cautery. In my seventeen years of treating more than 22,000 babies, I've had to use cautery only nine times. There is always the possibility of regrowth, but gentle stretching of the incision site for the first four to seven days prevents it. If regrowth happens, repeated cutting isn't necessary, because the tissue can easily be stretched open in the office.

Lasers are gaining popularity, more from marketing than anything else. They are generally performed by dentists who already have lasers and need a reason to use them. No one would go out and buy a laser to do frenulectomies. Lasers are also quite expensive for you and not covered by insurance. In my opinion, the only benefit of using a laser is that you don't have to see blood. But there are so many downsides, I worry that babies are suffering unnecessarily for huge profit margins.

Lasers cause tremendous pain and tissue damage. They also cut based on time, so the longer the dentist holds the laser in place, the deeper the cut. You baby won't nurse right away after the procedure. He will suffer two weeks of pain, and nursing will get worse before it gets better. Because lasers use heat to cut, there is more thermal damage, which results in more scarring and a longer healing time. You will have to stretch and tear incision sites aggressively to break up the scar tissue as it is forming. There is also a risk of cornea damage during the procedure, so everyone in the room needs to wear eye protection. Your baby has to be taken from you and held, or even tied down, so he doesn't move. Most parents aren't even allowed in the room when it's done. The sad part is that most parents don't realize that these horrible aspects of the procedure aren't necessary. They are even told to expect them. Even if the laser ends up helping a baby latch, this is huge price to pay—emotionally and literally. Some babies undergo repeated procedures, and when nursing doesn't improve, the dentist blames the mom.

You don't have to treat every baby who has gape restriction with a procedure. If you have a huge supply you can still nurse a little as long as it doesn't hurt, and pump to keep your supply up. You can also use a nipple shield if your baby can't latch on. Again, you have to also pump, because your baby won't be able to pull out the milk on her own. She will be able to get only what your breasts give her. Some moms are able to nurse like this for many, many months. But no one can tell you how long you will be able to maintain your supply, because none of these options fixes your baby's inability to efficiently transfer milk. You can forgo nursing and just pump and bottle-feed. Because gape restriction without tongue tie affects feeding only in the first year, *not* doing frenulectomies won't impact your baby in any other way unless she has a real tongue tie.

HOW GAPE RESTRICTION AND TONGUE TIE AFFECTS BOTTLE-FEEDING

Although most babies with gape restriction are able to bottle-feed, a high palate and set-back jaw may still cause issues. Because babies with gape restriction can't form a seal on bottle nipples, milk often leaks out the sides. These babies also swallow more air because of the extra space in their high palate. Some can't reach their tongue high enough to even compress the bottle nipple. They have to rely on gravity and often choke on the milk. If your baby's palate is high enough, the bottle nipple may not even touch her palate, so her suck reflex won't be triggered.

Babies that have a hard time bottle-feeding are sometimes diagnosed with low muscle tone. But the problem may be that her palate is too large for the bottle nipple. You may go through a whole slew of nipples but have only marginal improvement. No nipples are perfect, because they will all be too small for her mouth.

Some babies can't breast- or bottle-feed at all because of the severity of their gape restriction. In these cases, they have trouble feeding and gaining weight no matter what you do. Releasing the lip and tongue frenula in these babies is often the only solution, but they may need other supportive help.

SUCCESS RATES AND ALTERNATIVES

If you decide to do a procedure, you should understand that no procedure is risk-free. While cutting the upper and lower frenula always releases gape restriction, it doesn't necessarily *fix* breastfeeding. Even after frenulectomies, sometimes nursing improves only a little. I've even had babies refuse to nurse altogether after procedures. There are so many other factors involved, you have to consider all of them before deciding whether to move forward:

1. **AGE OF BABY:** While there isn't a cutoff age for performing these procedures, the longer a baby has nursed with gape restriction, the more variables there are to contend with. Your baby may have learned that

it's hard to get the milk out and developed different sucking behaviors, like clicking her tongue forward instead of pulling it back. She may get frustrated and distracted more easily. It's also harder to get an older baby to do what you want, so certain nursing positions are challenging. The bigger the baby, the heavier she is, which also affects your ability to hold her head and support your breast while nursing. In general, there is more variable improvement after three months. After six months, the chances fall even further.

2. **LOW MILK SUPPLY:** Even if you release your baby's gape, she won't want to nurse if she doesn't get a reward for her work. If you have a low supply, be prepared to supplement. Similarly, if it's later in the game (like eight to ten weeks) and your supply is dropping, getting her to latch more deeply will help her pull out what you have. It isn't likely to bring your whole supply back.

3. **NIPPLE AVERSION:** Once your baby learns that your breasts don't deliver, she will remember. She won't understand that once her frenula have been released, nursing will be easier. She will have to be convinced. All that convincing can create a lot of frustration for you and your baby. Some babies are so smart they become stubborn and refuse to nurse no matter what you do. You can fix the underlying gape problem, but you still have to fix the behavior. If this happens, see Chapter 13 for suggestions.

When I first started in ear, nose, and throat practice after residency, I joined a group of male doctors in a fancy Upper East Side office. They drew in a lot of patients, many of whom were babies with tongue tie who had trouble nursing. Although I had never heard of tongue tie, I quickly learned everything I could. Fueled by my own breastfeeding failure, I wanted to help moms avoid what I had endured. I also assumed tongue tie was something I should have learned in residency, and I was too embarrassed to ask for help.

Fast-forward a couple of years. I was treating more newborns with frenulectomies than anyone in Manhattan. I tried to convince my colleagues to learn how to do it. "Think of all the babies and moms you could help," I would say. But my pleading fell on deaf ears. One male colleague refused to learn, saying ear, nose, and throat had nothing to do with breasts. Another insisted he could figure out how to do these procedures on his own. He insisted that the tongue was there only to "tickle the nipple" and couldn't possibly be causing problems. Even my bosses were skeptical. One called me into his office to give me a lesson on tongue tie and told me I was doing unindicated procedures. But the proof was in the pudding. Baby after baby came in with problems and left nursing beautifully.

After the practice I worked for dissolved, I started my own practice and continued treating newborns with breastfeeding issues. There were a tiny number of lactation consultants in my inner circle. Together we formed a sort of underground breastfeeding network. We shared insights. They visited my office and shadowed me with patients. I spoke at their conferences. We even defended one another from pediatricians who warned moms against our advice and talked them out of the procedures.

It was during this time, because of all the success we had, that lactation consultants started branching out. I was only one doctor, so there was no way I could see everyone from the tristate area. They started referring moms and babies to local dentists and doctors for easier accessibility. The only problem was, these other practitioners knew very little about breastfeeding. Now there are so many people doing procedures, with no consistent protocols, that moms are left with a mixed bag of confusing advice. They don't know whom to believe.

Doctors have licenses, but no formalized teaching to learn how and why to do frenulectomies. At least ear, nose, and throat doctors are surgeons, so we can manage complications. Pediatricians and family practice doctors are not trained in sterile practice, and they aren't usually comfortable doing procedures. How dentists got into the mix is beyond me, but they have zero training in breastfeeding. They also don't take insurance for doing laser frenulectomies, so there is no regulatory oversight for what they are doing or claiming. Because dentists are cash based and in private practice, no one is watching them. At least in medicine there are grand rounds in hospital departments at which we have to report complications. There are also insurance companies monitoring our work. But not so in dentistry. A dentist can literally do whatever he wants unless someone complains. How can you complain if no one knows what standard practice is?

From the medical perspective, the practitioner performing a procedure has a moral and legal obligation to do no harm. This includes being able to give real informed consent for surgeries, large and small. We also have to be accountable for the outcomes of procedures. Somehow, moms have been made to believe that the person performing the frenulectomy is not responsible for supporting breastfeeding afterward. Even in my practice, after I've treated babies, moms often don't think to follow up with me if there is a problem. They go to a lactation consultant who wasn't in the office and has no idea what I did.

The sad part is that moms have a hard time finding anyone to listen and be willing to help with breastfeeding. When they do, it's even harder to know whom to trust. When you are desperate to breastfeed, you are easy to take advantage of. You will do almost anything to nurse your baby, and practitioners know that. A whole industry has been built around breastfeeding failure. When you're a new mom, you're at the mercy of practitioners who give adamant advice and perform procedures for things they often know nothing about. It's important to do your research. You are your baby's best advocate.

When choosing a practitioner to perform frenulectomies, here are some things to think about. While you may not find all the answers, you should at least be asking these questions:

1. What kind of help does the practitioner offer after the procedure? Are they motivated to help nursing or motivated to bill for the procedure?

2. Do they do procedures on every baby that comes in? How do they decide who is a good candidate?

3. What are their success rates? How can they show you, other than what they claim? Who referred you, and are they getting compensated for the referral?

4. What is their reputation in the community? How are they described in online groups?

5. How long have they been working with breastfeeding moms? Do they specialize in breastfeeding?

6. What kind of specific training have they done?

7. Are they a doctor or dentist?

8. How much surgical training have they had? Do they know how to deal with adverse outcomes?

9. Is the doctor male or female? If he is male, can he help you latch your baby on to nurse? How will he know the procedure worked? If the procedure doesn't work, how will he be able to assess it?

10. If the procedure doesn't work, what other sort of support can they offer?

If you ask these questions and don't like the answers, it's okay to get other opinions. It's also okay to avoid procedures altogether. But at least you'll be able to make an informed decision, so you're not led down a road of promises and deceit.

Weapons of Mass Lactation:
Issues with Milk Supply

Your supply is as individual as you are. We talk about low and normal supply and oversupply as if there are three categories, but supply is really a spectrum. You can fit anywhere on it. Some moms produce milk like a wall tap, while others can barely squeeze out a few drops. No one knows why some produce more than others.

While most moms make an average supply, the sad but honest truth is that not every mom will be able to make enough milk for her baby. Your being promised otherwise is outdated, patronizing, and just plain wrong. I understand where those promises come from—a desire to support every woman in her breastfeeding journey. But you deserve more than coddling and cheerleading. Denial doesn't help anyone. For some, low supply is medical and anatomic, but mostly it's because something went wrong in the first four to six weeks.

As we've discussed, the volume of milk your breasts can make is hormonally regulated. It also depends on the amount of glandular tissue in each breast and how fast your breasts make milk. We've already discussed how your baby's ability to transfer out milk with a deep latch affects your supply. But there are other ways to manipulate your supply with pumping and supplements if your baby isn't able to do it. And, like everything else in breastfeeding, timing is critical.

In this chapter we will look at the designations of *low supply* and *oversupply* and how having a supply at either end of the spectrum can affect your ability to nurse. I will explain how to tell if you are at risk of low supply and how medical conditions and your anatomy can contribute to it. I will also discuss the nebulous diagnosis of oversupply, how it affects your breastfeeding relationship, and suggestions for managing it. We will go over supplements and medications that alter your supply (up or down) and how pumping can help manage both.

Low Supply

Low supply is defined as anything less than what your baby needs. It can be a little as 1 to 2 ounces in a whole day or as much as 26 ounces a day. While the amount of milk you make is a moving target for the first month, from five weeks on, you should be able to make 28 to 32 ounces a day consistently. As your milk is coming in, it's hard to know if you will ultimately be able to make enough milk. But, as I covered in earlier chapters, you can look for clues that things are moving in the right direction. Your breasts should get engorged for the first few days. Milk should leak from them. Your baby should seem full after nursing ten to fifteen minutes on each side every two to three hours, and you should be able to pump at least 3 ounces from both breasts every two to three hours by five weeks. With all this milk, your baby should gain weight. If these things don't happen, you may have a low supply.

Although the supply-and-demand nature of your supply makes it hard to know for sure if you're able to make enough milk, the good news is that inherently low supply is very rare. In other words, the vast majority of moms will be able to make enough milk as long as things are going as they should. If you nurse with pain, your baby isn't emptying your breasts, and you aren't pumping to make up for it, you may lose a supply that could have otherwise been normal given the right circumstances. Low supply also runs in families, so ask your female relatives about their experiences nursing. If your baby is premature, your hormones may not have had time to catch up, so your supply may still be able to come in.

If your baby isn't gaining weight from nursing or is increasingly fussy at the breast, it's important to figure out if he has a shallow latch or you just have a low supply. It may even be both, because they go hand in hand. Don't assume everything will be fine if you have reason to believe otherwise. The difference is that a shallow latch is usually painful, and after you nurse for ten to fifteen minutes, you will be able to pump out more milk if you have a normal supply. If you have a low supply, there will be no milk to pump out.

Low supply doesn't mean you can't breastfeed. Even if you can't make a full supply, you can still give your baby what you make. Breastfeeding isn't all or none. Here are some disorders that cause inherently low supply:

1. **HYPOPLASIA**—Hypoplasia, or *insufficient glandular tissue (IGT),* basically means you have very little breast tissue. Even if your baby has a good latch, you will never have enough milk-making tissue to have a decent supply. If you have IGT, your breasts are different sizes. They are also widely spaced on your chest, and your areolae are large—sometimes the same size as your breasts. Some moms have stretch marks on their breasts despite their small size. With IGT, your breasts won't grow much during pregnancy or get engorged. Studies have shown that 85 percent of moms with IGT make less than half the milk their baby needs. This doesn't mean you can't nurse. It just means you should have realistic expectations and be even more vigilant in the first few weeks.

2. **BREAST SURGERY**—Breast surgery can be cosmetic (making them bigger or smaller) or medical (tumor removal, breast cancer). If you have implants, you won't automatically make less milk, especially if the implant was placed under your pectoralis muscle. But if you also have underlying IGT, you still won't have enough glandular tissue. If you had surgery to make your breasts smaller, you will obviously have less milk-making tissue, but it shouldn't make a huge difference in your supply. If you still have good blood flow and sensation, you should be fine. An incision that looks like a lollipop (around your nipple and straight down the middle of the underside of your breast) means your

surgeon did a good job. Similarly, if you had a tumor removed, the amount of breast tissue removed is important. Even if you had a whole breast removed, the other breast can often make up the difference.

3. **HORMONAL CAUSES**—Your supply is laid down and maintained by your hormones, so anything affecting your hormones can lower your ability to make milk. The most common hormonal causes of low supply are

   a. polycystic ovary disease
   b. hypothyroidism
   c. insulin-dependent diabetes—low insulin results in low milk production
   d. eating disorders

4. **OBESITY**—Obesity is often caused by the hormonal disorders mentioned above. As such, if your BMI is over 30, you may have a harder time converting breast tissue into milk-making tissue. Your prolactin levels may also be lower in the first week, so breastfeeding will be more challenging.

5. **TRAUMA AND RADIATION**—Anything that damages your breasts can make it harder to make milk.

PUMPING METHODS FOR LOW SUPPLY

Having a medical reason for low supply doesn't mean you should give up on breastfeeding. The same goes for losing your supply because you didn't realize things weren't going well in the first month or two. Depending on the kind of experience you want to have, you can still give your baby breastmilk. The good news is, because there are so many variables to milk production, you can pump in a certain way to increase, or at least maximize, what you have. Here are some things to consider:

Stronger vacuums are better than average ones.

One feature of modern pumps is different vacuum patterns. They start out with faster, softer suction, then switch to a slower and deeper rhythm after the first thirty seconds. This pattern is supposed to simulate your baby's mouth. Warming the flanges also increases the amount of milk that comes out in the first five minutes of pumping. You can also use a warm compress and hand stimulation to help your letdown. The best way to pull out as much milk as possible is with the highest vacuum you can tolerate comfortably.[1]

The way you pump—ten to fifteen minutes with full emptying and enough time between pumps for your breasts to fill up again—affects your total amount of milk.[2]

There is a lot of debate about how long you should pump when trying to maximize your supply. I've had moms tell me they were told to pump for an hour at a time, ten times a day. I appreciate the dedication, but it's not the suction that stimulates milk production. It's the milk removal. If there isn't any milk to remove, what's the point? If you remember the math, nearly half the milk in your breasts is removed during your first letdown. Even if you make milk quickly, you still have to give your breasts time to fill up again. For most moms, and especially if you have a low supply, most of your milk will be pulled out after the first eight to ten minutes.

Conversely, if you are trying to ramp up your supply, you can't just pump every few hours. If you go for longer stretches, like four to six hours, your supply will continue to go down. You can't pump for a few minutes a few times a day and expect to maintain or increase your supply. You have to completely empty your breasts each time.

Ideally, if you have a low supply, you should use your baby and the pump to maximize what you make. An example of one nursing regimen is to nurse for five to ten minutes on each side, followed by pumping for ten minutes (on each side or simultaneously) and then repeating the whole thing two hours later. That would be about ten sessions a day. You could do slightly more or less and see what works best for you. Some moms have a low storage capacity but they make milk quickly, so they can pump more often and end up with more total milk for the day. Find your sweet spot by keeping track of how much you get each time you pump. You can also work with a lactation consultant, some of whom specialize in pumping. Listening to calm music, looking at a picture of your baby, or holding him also helps your letdown.

Pumping both breasts is faster and doesn't hurt your supply.

A group of researchers at the University of Western Australia studied pumping dynamics in women who had normal supplies. They showed that pumping both breasts at the same time stimulated more letdowns, so it made the whole process go faster.[3] But it still removed the same percentage of milk as doing one breast at a time. Now most modern electrical pumps do both breasts simultaneously.

When you try to nurse, consider using a supplemental nursing system to supplement your low supply.

See Chapter 13 for details.

Whatever you decide, your pumping/nursing routine should never take precedence over bonding with your baby.

If it all feels like too much work for the few ounces of milk you make a day, it may be better to spend that time in other ways. Yes, breastmilk is amazing, but whole generations of people have survived without it. Do what's best for *both* you and your baby.

DRUGS TO INCREASE YOUR SUPPLY

Drugs to increase your supply are controversial. In the past, moms have been given everything from antipsychotics to hormones to try to get that prolactin going. Besides the obvious fear of side effects to the baby, these treatments were also not so great for moms. There was hope in nasal oxytocin spray, but it didn't work well. Other hormones have been tried, but ended up being expensive failures.

Although the idea of giving drugs to increase supply may sound sketchy, there is one drug that has been widely used all over the world. It is called domperidone. Originally formulated to calm upset stomachs and prevent nausea and vomiting, the pro-breastfeeding aspect was a side effect. Domperidone blocks dopamine, which just happens to raise prolactin levels.[4] I'm sure that didn't excite the people taking it for their gut, but it also proved dangerous for other reasons. When it was given intravenously to older, very sick cancer patients, it caused deadly heart arrhythmias.[5,6] In research mice, it also caused breast tumors when it was given for long periods of time.[7] A drug called Reglan is similar to domperidone but less effective at increasing milk production. It also has a higher chance of side effects.

Despite these issues, domperidone was approved by Health Canada more than twenty years ago. It was available over the counter in the UK until 2014, when the European Medicines Committee found that it caused a small increased risk of side effects in people over sixty with heart problems who took doses greater than 30 milligrams a day. In the United States, domperidone's use is limited. The FDA issued a warning in 2004, making it impossible to get from regular pharmacies. It was still available in compounding pharmacies until 2014, when the FDA went after them too. While it is legal for an American doctor to prescribe it, it is hard to find a local pharmacy that carries it. Most moms get it from Canada, provided it is for personal use, accompanied by a doctor's prescription and letter of necessity, and is for only a three-month supply.

The surprising thing about the domperidone controversy is that it has never caused problems in breastfeeding moms. Dr. Jack Newman, a Canadian pediatrician, is a huge proponent, and has been prescribing it since 1985. If it is given to moms who don't have a history of heart problems, it has been shown (at least anecdotally) to be pretty safe. However, because of ethical reasons, no studies have been done to prove its safety.

Unfortunately, because it is the only drug known to increase milk production, we are left in limbo.

Different dosing regimens can be used based on your situation. You should never take domperidone if you have a heart arrhythmia. If you have any history of heart disease, you should work with a doctor. The starting dose is usually 10 milligrams three times a day and goes up from there. It's best to start taking it within the first month of nursing, because that's when prolactin is most impactful. You should notice an increase in supply within the first three to seven days with a peak somewhere between two and four weeks. The recommended course is six weeks, but some moms need to continue past that to keep their supply going. The results are variable, and it doesn't work for everyone, so speak to your doctor before considering domperidone.

SUPPLEMENTS TO INCREASE YOUR SUPPLY

As I've said before, moms are resourceful. Just because no one in the medical world has figured out a way to increase supply safely doesn't mean moms will just give up. There are whole compendiums of ayurvedic herbs to support nursing. There are also foods and supplements called *galactagogues* that promote milk supply. Many were discovered because they help animals, like cows and goats, make more milk. I kid you not. Because supplements aren't technically drugs, the FDA may issue safety profiles but doesn't regulate them.

Regardless of the cause of your low supply, galactagogues can be helpful, but only if you empty your breasts completely and regularly while taking them. If you don't, you can get engorgement, plugged ducts, and mastitis, or they won't make a difference. In some cultures, moms start taking them right after birth anyway. There have been few studies to prove their benefit.[8] There also aren't "proven" doses, so the recommended dose is kind of a guess. Even though they are over the counter, you still have to make sure they are safe for you. Some have side effects. Also, keep in mind that many over-the-counter teas or preparations often have a combination of different supplements. Read the labels and consult with your doctor first.

1. **FENUGREEK:** This herb with seeds tastes like maple syrup. It has been touted to have many medical benefits, such as for digestive problems, painful menstruation, polycystic ovary syndrome (PCOS), and kidney issues. It comes in tea or supplements. There have been a couple of recent studies showing that it can significantly increase milk production, but no one knows why.[9] The best guess is that it acts like plant-based estrogen. Fenugreek is not safe if you have thyroid issues of any kind or if you are taking blood thinners. Common side effects are stomach upset and maple-smelling urine.

2. **GALEGA (GOAT'S RUE):** Used for centuries to increase breastmilk and aid in diabetes, for moms with IGT and PCOS, but no one knows how it works. Because it can lower blood sugar levels, watch for hypoglycemia and don't take it if you are diabetic.

3. **SILYMARIN (MILK THISTLE):** The active substance in milk thistle, silymarin is mainly used to support the liver, but it also may stimulate estrogen receptors. It is generally considered safe if you take the recommended dose. Side effects, like nausea, diarrhea, bloating, or itching, are rare.

4. **SHATAVARI (WILD ASPARAGUS):** This has been used as in India for centuries to support female reproductive conditions like PCOS, as well as depression and anxiety. It is included in the official ayurvedic pharmacopoeia for normalizing lactation. It has very few side effects, but some people are allergic to it.

5. **TORBANGUN, OR COLEUS AMBOINICUS LOUR ("MEXICAN MINT"):** This herb has been used for hundreds of years in Indonesia to promote milk production. Several studies have proven its benefits without side effects. It is also used for cough, bronchitis, and diarrhea.

6. **OATMEAL:** While there is no downside to eating oatmeal, no research has proven that it increases milk supply. Also, no one knows the mechanism of how it works or if steel-cut oats are better than rolled oats. Many "lactation cookies" are made of oatmeal.

7. **BEER:** Used for centuries to increase breastmilk in moderate amounts, the surprise is that it's not the alcohol that does it. It's the barley that stimulates prolactin. Nonalcoholic beers with just plain barley are just as good.

Oversupply

Oversupply is defined as a faster-than-usual letdown, increased flow, a huge volume of milk, or a combination of all three. Oversupply may seem like a champagne problem, especially to moms who struggle with supply, but it's really a mixed bag. No one knows why some moms make more milk than others, but we can make some guesses. The foundational cause is likely hormonal, like having too much prolactin that converts breast tissue to milk-making alveoli. You can also increase an already ample supply by pumping more often. Some moms produce endless milk no matter what they do. My guess is they lack FIL (feedback inhibitor of lactation) so their breasts don't have a stopgap, but no one has proven this. If we could figure out why some moms make so much milk, maybe we could better help moms with low supply. For now, that's just an idea for future research.

The term *oversupply* can be misleading because it assumes having a lot of milk is a problem. In truth, it depends on the situation. If you are a mom who has a huge supply and your baby can latch deeply, you may not run into problems. Conversely, if your baby has a shallow latch and can't manage your supply, you may be labeled as having an oversupply but it's really your baby's anatomy that's the problem. Before you assume it's you, check your baby's gape and latch. If you correct his gape, your "oversupply" may become a good thing. To make sense of this, let's take a more granular look at what's happening.

If you have a huge supply, it's obvious. You will leak milk

between feedings, have frequent engorgement and plugged ducts, and feel overfull a lot of the time. Your baby may struggle to drink from the wall tap that is your flow, sputtering and choking to keep up. When you have a lot of milk, the sugary foremilk floats to the surface, so your baby gets that first. If you remember, the fatty part of your milk is what makes him feel full and fall asleep. So, when he only gets sugary milk, he will want to eat all the time and will gain a lot of weight quickly. He may also have green, explosive stools and get colic and gas.

A baby's latching problems are often missed if you have an oversupply. If you have nipple pain and your baby takes a long time to nurse, it may seem like everything is okay because he is gaining weight. But if you look only at weight gain as a measure of normal breastfeeding, you can miss the boat and run into trouble later. Moms with huge supplies often suffer more because no one pays attention to their symptoms. This isn't only bad for you. It also means your baby is struggling with his latch.

Just because you make a lot of milk at first, it doesn't mean you will be able to keep making a lot of milk if your baby isn't latched correctly. A big supply can mask your baby's latching problems early on. Then, somewhere between six and ten weeks in, things can change. Your baby will get fussy at the breast, and your supply can drop suddenly. This happens because after that amount of time, your supply is more closely regulated by FIL. If your breasts haven't been getting emptied regularly, they fill up less each time you nurse. Over time, your supply goes down. It's harder to bring back a supply once it drops, so don't ignore symptoms of a shallow latch just because your baby is gaining weight. Don't nurse through the pain.

EMPTYING TO MANAGE OVERSUPPLY

Getting the right ebb and flow can be challenging with a huge supply. On the one hand, you need to empty your breasts often to prevent engorgement. But if you empty your breasts too often, you can increase an otherwise huge supply. The key is getting creative with timing your pumping and emptying. It is helpful to work with a lactation consultant when managing an oversupply. If you can't afford one or don't have access, try these recommendations:

1. Fully empty both breasts by pumping both sides simultaneously for 15 minutes first thing in the morning.

2. An hour later, *block feed*—this means nursing on one breast for 15 minutes, waiting 2 to 3 hours, then nursing on the other side for 15 minutes, waiting 2 hours, back to side one, and so on.

3. If you get too full in the middle of the day, do another power pump on both sides.

4. Store extra milk in the fridge or freezer, and/or consider donating to a local milk bank.

- Pump out the initial letdown for 5 minutes before nursing.
- Use the laid-back position so your baby can nurse against gravity (pages 118, 119–20).
- After your baby nurses, use a hand or electric pump to empty plugged ducts.

Medications and Drugs That Affect Supply

Your supply can be affected in either direction by medications or other drugs. Some of these medications are necessary for health reasons, but most are optional. If you want to keep nursing, you should avoid those that block milk production so they don't sabotage your supply. The supplements I already mentioned can help bring back your supply if you accidentally take something that hurts it. If you have too much milk or want to stop nursing, there are medications to regulate that as well.

- *Alcohol:* A little alcohol is okay. But if you drink a lot of alcohol and try to nurse, not only will it make your baby drunk, but it will also prevent your brain from releasing oxytocin.
- ***Decongestants that contain pseudoephedrine:*** Pseudoephedrine is found in all kinds of over-the-counter decongestants. When you reach for cold relief, make sure you check the labels. When combined with antihistamines, its effect can be even

worse. A single dose can cause an immediate drop in your production by decreasing prolactin in your blood. If you keep taking it, you can lose your supply altogether, and it's hard to bring it back. Moms who are trying to reduce their supply often try pseudoephedrine, but it's hard to know how much each dose will affect your supply. I suggest working with your OB/GYN or a lactation consultant before trying this on your own.

- *Birth control:* Although breastfeeding is supposed to be a natural contraceptive, some moms want the extra assurance. Estrogen, one hormone used for birth control, prevents your brain from releasing prolactin. It can affect your supply, especially if you take it early on. Copper IUDs without hormones are another option.

- *Nicotine:* Whether you smoke or use a patch, nicotine lowers your prolactin. It also isn't safe for your baby, causing damage to his heart and lungs. Avoid it at all costs.

- *Herbs:* Sage, jasmine, peppermint, and parsley in large amounts are thought to lower your supply. You can use them to regulate your supply if you make too much milk, but you should avoid them if you struggle with supply. Sometimes they are buried in prepared foods, so check your labels!

- *Bromocriptine and ergotamine*: These medicines, used for migraines, reduce prolactin for eight to twelve hours with each dose. In the past they were used to stop lactation in moms who didn't want to breastfeed, but now they are banned because they can also hurt your heart.[10]

- *Methergine:* This drug is used to shorten labor and reduce blood loss, so you may not know if it was given to you. If your milk isn't coming in right away, ask if you were given this drug, as it decreases your supply. It also isn't safe for your baby for the first twelve hours, so you should pump and dump.

- *Diuretics:* Drugs like Lasix and hydrochlorothiazide are used for high blood pressure and heart problems that cause a backup of blood in your body. If you are given these drugs, there is probably a really good medical reason and it's likely you can't stop taking them. But be aware that high doses can also decrease your supply.

- *Antidepressants:* Common antidepressants, such as Prozac, Zoloft, and Lexapro, are selective serotonin reuptake inhibitors (SSRIs). They prevent your brain from reabsorbing serotonin and producing more of it. They may also delay your ability to lay down a supply in the first few days. If you need to go back on medication for your mental health, there is the option of breastfeeding or pumping for just a few weeks.

Feeding Frenzy: *What Abnormal Nursing Is Telling You*

When you become a new mom, you have to learn a new language. In lieu of words, your baby uses her cry to tell you what she needs. She also has behaviors based on reflexes and new ones she learns when those reflexes don't get her what she needs. Personality comes into play too. Even if you have other children, you can't always rely on past experiences to interpret your new baby. You are left responding to what you think your baby needs, discovering if you were right or wrong only after the fact.

How do you make sense of your baby's cries and cues? You can try listening to her, figuring out what she's trying to say through trial and error. Or you can read the customized manual that comes out with your placenta. That's a joke, of course, but wouldn't it be great? It's never that easy. Like many things in life, the test comes before the lesson. Understanding your baby takes time and patience. But there are some shared behaviors that tell you something is wrong. Sadly, because these behaviors are so common, many of them have been pulled into the spectrum of normal when they really are a literal cry for help. These problems can be complex, with more than one cause. They should be broken down and understood, not normalized.

In this chapter, I will explain these behavior patterns to help speed up your learning curve. A lot of this information was covered in previous chapters, but here I'm putting it into context so you can have it all in one place. Not every problem is fixable, but it's better to understand what's happening so you can address the real problem and stop blaming yourself. With these insights, you'll be speaking baby in no time.

Dry Diapers

If your baby isn't making enough wet diapers, it means she isn't taking in enough milk. The question is why? If you are exclusively breastfeeding, you have to figure out if it's your supply or her inability to transfer out your milk, or both.

The expected number of wet diapers by age is as follows:

- *Day 1:* first wet diaper by 12 to 24 hours
- *Day 2:* two wet diapers a day
- *Day 3 to 5:* three to five wet diapers a day
- *Day 6 and on:* six to eight wet diapers a day

If your baby is under one month, figuring out your supply can be a moving target, as we discussed in Chapter 11. In the first week, it is common for your baby to lose weight and have dry diapers while your supply moves from colostrum to transitional milk. But your supply could also be inherently low (meaning you can't make much milk no matter what you do). If that's the case, you won't have engorgement or leaking, your breasts may look smaller and widely spaced, and, even when you pump, you won't get much. Although it's rare, it's pretty obvious early on if you have inherently low supply. While you figure it out, it's a good idea to supplement with formula or donor milk right away. If your baby is losing too much weight, you need to feed her while you figure out the problem.

If you have early indicators of a good supply that then dwindles, it means your baby isn't transferring out your milk. Note whether you have pain when you nurse. Check for a restricted gape and shallow latch. Look for an obvious tongue tie. Check her palate to see if it is high and arched and if her chin is recessed. Look for a blister on her upper lip. If she has transfer problems, consider an intervention or just pump and bottle-feed to keep your supply going.

Babies who have trouble transferring milk from a bottle are a special case. See the section on prolonged feeding (page 205) for more details.

Weight Loss or Slow Gain

It's normal for your baby to lose 7 to 10 percent of her birth weight in the first week, but she should regain it within the first two weeks. After the first week, she should gain as follows:

- $^2/_3$ to 1 ounce (19 to 28 grams) a day
- 4 to 7 ounces (.25 to .5 lb, or 112 to 200 g) a week
- 32 ounces (2 lbs or 0.9 kg) a month

Even if your baby isn't gaining as expected, there is a wide range of normal. That's why there is a growth curve. If she is on the curve but not headed in the right direction, don't fall prey to wishful thinking. True, the growth curve is a range, but falling within the curve alone isn't enough. If your baby starts off in the upper range and drops to a lower range, something is wrong. Also pay attention to her patterns of weight gain or loss. If she starts out with low weight and skyrockets, she could be dealing with a huge supply with or without a shallow latch.

Causes for weight loss or slow gain are similar to causes for dry diapers. If she is not gaining, it is because you have a low supply, she is not transferring milk, or a combination of both. If you figure out that your supply is the problem, you can adjust your feeding and pumping schedule and start taking supplements. But if you have an inherently low supply, you have to supplement to make up the difference. It doesn't mean you have to stop nursing.

Sometimes weight loss or slow gain is because of your baby's transfer issues. In addition to tongue tie and shallow latch, ask your doctor or lactation consultant to check for low muscle tone. You can tell the difference because low muscle tone doesn't cause pain, but nursing and the others usually do. Sometimes babies don't gain weight because they won't wake up to nurse or because they are premature, etc. Others want to eat all the time and never seem satisfied. In order to figure out cause and effect, you should look at her behavior as a whole.

Prolonged Nursing with
Falling Asleep at the Breast

After the first week, it should take your baby ten to fifteen minutes of nursing on each breast to get enough milk to fall asleep for two to three hours. This is a general rule and mostly meant as a reference. While baby-led nursing is popular and usually the goal, you can't always follow your baby's needs, especially if she falls asleep or wants to nurse all the time. It may seem like letting her take an hour to nurse gets her more milk, but that isn't necessarily the case. If she is nursing efficiently, it shouldn't take her that long. Long nursing sessions mean she is working way too hard. It also means your breasts aren't getting emptied quickly and fully enough, so you could eventually lose your supply if you don't also pump. Don't assume your baby is "comfort feeding" if she nurses for fifty minutes, falls asleep, then wakes up crying when you try to take her off. While it is fine to nurse your baby to sleep on your breast, long nursing sessions where she isn't transferring milk are not a good thing. You can bond with your baby in other ways. Having your baby asleep on your breast can be comforting, but if she is passed out from exhaustion, it is not breast-feeding.

If your baby is premature, it is common for her to sleep a lot because her reflexes haven't "woken up" yet. You may have to pump and supplement her with a bottle for the first few days or weeks until her gape reflex kicks in. Full-term babies are sometimes sleepy too. Things like delivery method, compression on their upper spine from a prolonged vaginal birth, sitting in a fixed position for most of the pregnancy, or birth trauma can blunt their root, gape, and suck reflexes. If you are taking pain medication with opiates, it can transfer to your baby through your breastmilk. Even though your doctors may assure you it is fine, the drug will make your baby sleepy.

Low tone is very rare, and not the same as blunted reflexes. If your baby has it, she won't be able to generate enough muscle control to gape and latch on. She may even struggle with a bottle. Check her suck strength by having her suck on your finger. She should be able to form a seal around it that feels tight and firm. When you pull out your finger, you should feel like you are breaking a seal. You may even hear a pop. A baby with low tone will move her tongue around in a random way on the breast and the bottle. She also won't cause pain when she nurses. Usually babies outgrow low tone, but they may need feeding support until they do. Check with your pediatrician to be sure.

Sadly, sometimes babies may have neurological delay that becomes apparent because they have trouble feeding or nursing. These babies can't coordinate suck-swallow movements. They can't form a seal on a bottle or breast, and may not show any hunger cues at all. The whole process of feeding is hard no matter how they are fed. These cases are very rare and should be seen by a feeding specialist.

Before you decide whether your baby has low tone, feel the roof of her mouth (palate). If it feels high and arched or cupped—you can fit your fingertip into it—that could be the culprit. Sometimes babies who can't seem to coordinate their latch just have a high palate. Remember that the suck reflex is stimulated by pressing on the baby's palate. If the bottle nipple or your breast can't reach up that high, your baby won't suck. This may make it seem like she has low tone. Similar problems can occur with tongue tie or *cleft palate,* when the roof of her mouth doesn't close entirely. In both cases, her tongue can't reach up high enough to compress against the roof of her mouth.

Falling asleep at the breast and waking up for the bottle can be from low supply, a transfer issue, or both. The reason your baby falls asleep is because of our friend cholecystokinin. Remember that cholecystokinin is released in two ways. A small burst of it is released when your baby first latches on to calm her down so she can eat. If she gets milk, that cholecystokinin goes away and she will stay awake to keep nursing until the fat from your milk gets to her small intestine. When the fat fills her tummy, another, bigger burst of cholecystokinin is released, making her fall asleep for two to three hours. If your baby nurses and doesn't get milk, small bursts of cholecystokinin will keep getting released, and she will keep falling asleep at the breast. But when each small burst wears off, she will wake up hungry. Cholecystokinin makes her fall asleep to protect her from wasting energy when she isn't getting enough food.

Cluster Feeding

Cluster feeding is when your baby wants to nurse constantly in "clusters" of time. It is most common in the first few weeks, usually in the late afternoon or early evening. It happens so often that it has been normalized into something moms should expect. The long-held belief is that babies nurse around the clock because they are going through a growth spurt. While growth spurts do happen, there are other causes for cluster feeding. At its core, cluster feeding means your baby needs more milk than she is getting. True, babies don't always nurse in the cadence we expect. But there is a difference between your baby wanting to nurse frequently for a few days because she is growing and her wanting to nurse all the time because she isn't getting enough milk, period. To differentiate between the two, look at the whole picture. Most cluster feeding is usually the latter.

A common pattern of abnormal cluster feeding is a baby who sleepily nurses through the day, falls asleep at the breast, then suddenly wakes up late afternoon or early evening and goes to town, sometimes nursing for hours. Some babies sleep all day and nurse all night. If it happens for a few days, fine. But if this is your regular feeding pattern or it happens for weeks, there is a problem with milk transfer, your supply, or both. Usually, you have pain when your baby has a shallow latch, and unless you have an oversupply, she won't gain weight well. Assess yourself for low supply to see if the problem is your supply alone. Continuing to cluster feed with pain for weeks will also reduce an otherwise good supply, so take that into account.

Another cluster-feeding scenario happens when a baby struggles with a huge supply. This is a little different than the others because in this case, babies want to nurse all the time but they gain a lot of weight very quickly. Pediatricians will mistake this as being great if they care only about weight gain. But cluster feeding is not good for you or your baby. If you have a big supply, the sugary foremilk floats to the surface, and your baby gets that first. She may fill up on sheer volume of sugary milk before she even gets to the fatty hindmilk. This will make her fall asleep for a little while, then wake up hungry again because the fatty milk didn't create a huge surge of cholecystokinin to knock her out for a few hours. She will eat and eat and eat because her hunger cues aren't being regulated by your milk fat. It will be like she is on a high-carb diet, always chasing that next sugar high. To remedy this, try the pumping schedules recommended in Chapter 11, emptying some of the foremilk before she nurses.

Choking While Nursing

If your baby has a hard time managing the milk from your breast, it is usually because of high flow or volume when you have a huge supply. Most of the time, your baby will regulate your supply over the first few weeks. You can help her out with the pumping schedules mentioned in Chapter 11.

Choking on a huge supply doesn't necessarily mean it's all your supply's fault. Babies can struggle with a huge supply and be unable to regulate it if they have a shallow latch. If your baby can't unhinge her jaw to gape and form a seal, she will leak, sputter, and choke. If she can gape normally, she will eventually be able to control the flow. She does this by clenching down on your nipple in the back of her throat, protecting herself from getting waterboarded by all the milk. Check for a shallow latch and high palate before assuming the problem is only because of your huge supply.

Clicking on the Breast

When your baby can't latch deeply, she usually also has a hard time moving her tongue normally. This can be because of tongue tie or because her set-back jaw holds her tongue back. Normal tongue movement is to pull the tongue up to compress the breast against the palate, then back to extract milk from the nipple and down to swallow. Without that ability, your baby can learn to snap her tongue *forward* instead. This forward movement makes a clicking sound. Clicking always means your baby isn't latched deeply. You can try repositioning, but if she can't gape widely, she won't be able to latch deeply without an intervention.

Clicking also goes hand in hand with gas and colic because they stem from the same cause. If your baby undergoes a procedure, the clicking doesn't automatically stop. It can continue unless you compress her against the breast with her new latch, preventing her from doing it. Eventually, once your baby learns this deeper latch, she will stop clicking.

Refusing the Breast and Nipple Confusion

There are many ways your baby can refuse the breast. I like to divide breast refusal into three categories, with the first and last on either end of the spectrum.

- *The aloof baby:* Falls asleep at the very smell of you, anytime she gets near your breast.
- *The frantic baby:* Latches on like her life depends on it, sucks for a minute or two, then cries and goes on and off.
- *The angry baby:* Used to love to nurse, even for marathon sessions, and now cries when you try to latch her on, sometimes hitting or punching your breasts.

All three behaviors are your baby's way of telling you something is wrong. While it's easy to blame yourself, don't bother. Everyone else will. The irony is that breast refusal is almost never your fault. It's easy to ignore cues and patterns and follow wrong advice that gets you to breast refusal. But rather than get caught up in the blame game, let's review normal baby-to-breast behavior to understand what these breast refusal behaviors mean.

When your baby is ready to nurse, she should show early hunger cues, like turning toward your breast, being more awake, cooing, rooting, flexing her arms and legs, and putting her fingers and hands in her mouth. She should gape widely, latch on with a seal, and be able to pull milk out of your breasts without causing you pain.

Let's start with the aloof baby. This kind of breast refusal is the hardest to interpret because you have very little to go on. If your baby is premature, she may be sleepy because her gape reflex hasn't kicked in yet. Sometimes full-term babies also have a delay in reflexes, depending on how they were delivered.

Every once in a while, the refusal happens after a baby tries to latch a few times, doesn't get milk, then stops trying. Of course, her refusal will push you into giving her a bottle. She will continue with that bottle because she will quickly figure out that she can't get milk from your breasts.

The frantic baby is a different version of the aloof baby. This baby is panicked and wakes up screaming in hunger. She cries and cries until she latches and then sucks within an inch of her life. She may pass out after a few minutes, then wake up again, hungry and angry. If you nurse a frantic baby and she is still hungry afterward, try pumping out milk to see if you have any left. If you do, you likely have a normal supply but your baby isn't transferring milk. You can try giving her a bottle of formula or pumped milk, which she will probably gobble down, proving my point. If you don't have pain and never got engorged or leaked milk, the problem may be that you have a low supply. You should strongly consider supplementing while you figure everything out.

Frantic babies can also happen when moms have a huge supply. Just like cluster feeders, if you have a lot of milk and your baby can't transfer it out, she will be desperate to eat. She will try and try, pass out, and be gassy from getting only foremilk. When you offer her food from another source, she will hungrily eat it. This is because she is burning through the sugary foremilk and never feels full. She may also have gas and colic from the foremilk, which makes her want to eat more to calm down her tummy. Unfortunately, eating more foremilk only upsets her stomach more, so the cycle continues.

If you keep trying to nurse a frantic baby and follow up

your feeding session with a bottle, she will eventually become an angry baby. Angry babies are frantic babies who learned to associate your breasts with hunger and pain. Remember that your baby's sense of smell is very strong, and her connection to the waxy substance around your nipples is hardwired. Imagine what it is like for her to smell your breasts, latch on, suck and suck only to get very little milk, cry in hunger, and then get an easy-to-drink bottle. Over time, she will learn to associate your breasts with suffering and the bottle with relief. Angry babies are angry because they are working too hard for food and spending a lot of time feeling hungry. This would stress anyone out. And when you're the mom of an angry baby, you will get stressed out too. Here is where the paradox happens. Moms of angry babies are often blamed for their baby's anger when the opposite is true. Your stress doesn't hinder her reflexes. She is hangry. But when moms are made to feel guilty, they keep trying to make it better. Suffering is reinforced for both.

Which brings us to nipple confusion. I joke that nipple confusion isn't confusion at all. The baby knows exactly what's up. She learns to avoid the nipple when she doesn't get milk from it. Nipple aversion isn't something that happens randomly. It is trained into babies when moms follow well-meaning advice to keep nursing no matter what. Here's how it works.

You baby is hardwired to look for your breasts by smelling the waxy substance around your nipple. This makes her gape and latch. If she keeps trying and failing to gape and latch, she won't get enough milk, you will have pain, and both of you will be stressed out. Your baby will eventually turn into a frantic or angry baby, and you will be miserable. Once her weight starts dropping, you will have to explain the problem to your pediatrician. Because of the weight loss, you will be told to supplement with a bottle. Even though she prefers you, a hungry baby will eat from any food source. Here is where good intentions backfire. You will be told to keep nursing your frantic baby so she doesn't "forget" your breasts. Your baby won't forget your breasts. She is hardwired to want them. But if you repeatedly create an association of hunger and frustration with the smell of your breasts and follow that with the positive reinforcement of an outside food source, she will *learn* to choose the other source over you. Usually that source is a bottle, so bottles get blamed for nipple confusion, but other feeding sources, like the spoon, finger, cup, or syringe have the same effect. They may prevent bottle preference, but they won't prevent nipple aversion. Your baby will never inherently reject you. If she smells you and gets milk from your breasts, she will always prefer you. If she smells you and can't get milk, she will develop a negative association with you, sometimes as fast as Day 1.

If you want to avoid nipple aversion, it is best to pump and bottle-feed while deciding how to address milk-transfer issues or low supply. Chapter 13 will go over treatments for nipple aversion.

Reflux, Gas, and Colic

There is a range of reflux symptoms, from burping and farting (gas) to spitting up to colic, excessive pain, and weight loss. Seventy to 85 percent of babies have reflux symptoms during the first two months of life. By the time they are one year old, the symptoms mostly go away. The term *reflux* is misleading, however, because babies don't have much acid in their stomachs. They are still developing their microbiome with the help of your breastmilk, so reflux in a baby is not the same as reflux in an adult.

Your baby's digestive system starts getting colonized by bacteria in your womb. Bacteria continues to populate her gut based on the way she was born. Vaginal births populate her with the bacteria *Lactobacillus, Prevotella,* or *Sneathia,* while C-section births result in *Staphylococcus, Corynebacterium,* and *Propionibacterium.* During her first week, she will develop other bacteria, based on whether she is breast- or formula-fed. Taking antibiotics while breastfeeding can kill bacteria in her gut as well. Probiotics are not generally recommended in newborns.

It's easy to misread gas and colic cues unless you learn to understand your baby's cry. Crying from gas or colic is a painful cry. It comes on suddenly and can go on for hours. Gassy babies also arch their backs, kick or punch, and straighten out their legs. Nothing seems to console them, not even feeding or walking around. You can try laying them over your shoulder to burp them, but that alone rarely helps. Babies with a lot of gas get bad reputations as being fussy, while those that don't cry are labeled as "good." These labels aren't fair. You'd cry too if you were in pain all the time.

Spitting up occasionally is normal, but some babies projectile vomit across the room. If this happens, ask your pediatrician about a condition called *pyloric stenosis.* Pyloric stenosis is when the muscular portion of your baby's lower stomach becomes thickened and doesn't allow food to pass through. It can lead to dehydration and weight loss and is the second most common reason newborns need surgery.

Reflux, gas, and colic are a range of symptoms that stem from one of three main causes, or a combination of them:

1. You have a huge supply, so your baby is only getting sugary foremilk.
2. Something you are eating is getting through your milk and giving her gas.
3. She has a high palate and shallow latch and swallows air every time she nurses.

We've already discussed how your supply affects nursing in Chapter 11, so let's move on to how your diet affects her. Babies can have allergies or intolerances to certain foods. Allergies usually cause a rash and bloody stool. They can also cause wheezing, hives, vomiting, diarrhea, and a stuffy nose. The most common allergy is to cow's milk protein, which happens in up to half of babies with reflux or gas. Many foods are laced with dairy, so make sure to check labels. Other common culprits are eggs, corn, peanuts, soy, wheat/gluten, fish, sesame seeds, tree nuts, shellfish, mustard, and celery. Your baby can also have an intolerance to foods like broccoli, garlic, beans, onions, excess sugar, chocolate, and so on. Unlike allergies, food intolerance usually just ups her gas and spit-up but doesn't otherwise hurt her.

Hunting down the food culprit is tricky. It's good to keep a food journal and compare it to her symptoms. Her reactions can be delayed, however, sometimes popping up a few days to a several weeks later. Journals may not pinpoint the problem, but at least they can steer you in the right direction. You can also try an elimination diet, removing suspected foods. It's best to start eliminating the most common allergens, like dairy and soy. Remove each food protein one at a time. If the eliminated food is the problem, your baby's symptoms should improve in two to three days and resolve completely in a week. If you reintroduce the food, she will usually react within six hours. Your baby's reaction is also dose dependent, meaning the more of the food you eat, the worse the symptoms.

Perhaps the most common cause of reflux, gas, and colic in babies, and the most overlooked, is from cause number three: swallowing air while bottle- or breastfeeding. Your baby's high palate and shallow latch is usually the reason for this. Tongue tie and gape restriction, which go along with a high palate, prevent her from lifting her tongue high enough to compress the bottle or breast against the roof of her mouth. Every time she swallows, she takes down a big gulp of air. You can sometimes hear the air going down. On the bottle, milk will leak out the sides. Medications don't help because the problem is mechanical. The only way to make it better is to correct the latch or switch to a bottle nipple that fills the space. See Chapter 13 for more details.

Nipple Pain

I dedicated an entire chapter to breast and nipple pain, so I won't belabor it here. But as a quick summary:

Some mild pain when you first start nursing is common, but not all pain is the same. There is huge difference between discomfort and toe-curling agony. Nipple pain is caused by friction. Friction is caused by a restricted gape and shallow latch with or without tongue tie or from tongue tie alone. Restricted gape and tongue tie are anatomic problems that your baby is born with, which do not get better without intervention. If you have friction, you can also develop surface infections on your nipples, such as thrush (which is a fungal infection), or deeper infections in your breasts, such mastitis. Do not ignore nipple pain, because it is a warning that something is wrong with your baby's latch. Nipple pain can also lead to postpartum depression. If you suffer through it, the pain may go away, but not because the latch gets better. Your nipples suffer so much damage that they can become less sensitive and scarred.

Patient Perspective

Jennifer was a three-week-old baby who was diagnosed with tongue tie at birth by the lactation consultant in the hospital. A second lactation consultant agreed, but her pediatrician disagreed, saying the tongue tie was slight and didn't need addressing. Jennifer spent a couple of days in the NICU for observation and was given formula. Since then, her mom started breastfeeding, but she had been having a lot of nipple pain. It was so painful, she began dreading breastfeeding. She tried the side-lying nursing position because of her C-section incision, but it didn't help. She had been taking Percocet, but when she stopped, her nipple pain became more noticeable and severe. When Jennifer tried to latch, she couldn't open her mouth very wide, and she had a hard time latching and staying on the breast. She fed every two to three hours for thirty minutes and had some mild gas. She was gaining weight, but her mom was still able to pump three ounces out of her breasts even after Jennifer has finished nursing.

On exam, Jennifer had a normal frenulum with no tongue tie, a high-arched, cupped palate, and a set-back jaw. The baby underwent lip and tongue frenulectomies and was able to gape and latch immediately after the procedures. Mom was told to make a mixture of Monistat and Neosporin cream and apply it to her breasts after each feeding for the next few days to heal the nipple damage.

Torticollis

Torticollis is when one of your baby's neck muscles, the big muscle in the front and side of her neck called the *sternocleido-mastoid*, becomes shortened and tightened. If your baby has torticollis, she will keep her head turned to one side no matter what position you put her in. No one knows what causes torticollis, but it most likely happens because of the way your baby sits in your womb. If she is stuck in one position, her neck muscles grow in a particular way and then scar and harden.

Torticollis happens more often in firstborns. Babies with torticollis often also have hip dysplasia, when the bands that connect the muscles and bones of her hips are extra stretchy. Babies with torticollis also develop asymmetric jaws because bones are shaped by the way muscles pull them. For all these reasons, babies with torticollis can struggle to breastfeed. Treatment is with physical therapy and craniosacral therapy.

Mommy's Little Helpers:
Possible Interventions

I often joke that if men had to breastfeed, either everyone would have starved to death or someone would have figured out how to fix breastfeeding problems a thousand years ago. Men don't easily accept prolonged pain and suffering without giving up or doing something about it. But women are different. We can, and do, put up with almost anything. Especially when it comes to our babies. When breastfeeding sucks, we accept the confusing and often contradictory advice given by everyone from the labor and delivery nurse to the on-call pediatrician. Even well-meaning lactation consultants imply that breastfeeding failure is our fault. It's not just a problem with the healthcare providers. In some ways, we are our own worst enemies.

Moms derive meaning from martyrdom. We are primed even before giving birth to expect suffering. We are told that our nipples will hurt, bleed even, and we accept it. I mean, childbirth is painful, right? And we made it through that! We accept that blame, as if suffering makes us better moms. I can't tell you how many times moms I've seen in my office told me they felt selfish for wanting to breastfeed without suffering. I often have to convince moms that their suffering is unnecessary, and that it means their baby is suffering too.

The resistance to accepting help is also physiological. By the time a new mom has endured even a week of painful nursing, she is at risk of postpartum depression for up to six months after she *stops* nursing. Pain creates physiologic depression and a feeling of hopelessness. With too much cortisol and too little oxytocin, bonding is affected as well, creating even more shame and less desire to get help. Breastfeeding is your *reward* for giving birth. It may be rocky at times, but it's not supposed to be punishing.

Now that you have a better sense of your baby's red flags, let's talk about what to do about them. Most recommendations meant to support breastfeeding come from the perspective that anyone can nurse. Think back to our discussion of La Leche. This organization was founded during a time when moms were being steered away from breastfeeding for a whole host of reasons. From the La Leche perspective, anything challenging or limiting was washed over and pulled into the spectrum of normal. The goal was to make breastfeeding work no matter what. It was a good place to start, but we are a long way from the 1950s. That big push to save breastfeeding has swung to the other side of the pendulum. New moms today are told to breastfeed at any cost, without a real sense of what they are up against, and with outdated recommendations that sometimes make their suffering worse.

True, most moms can breastfeed. Some can do it on their

own, but most need help. Others won't be able to nurse without interventions, medications, or supplements. Some won't be able to nurse no matter what, either because of their own or their baby's medical or anatomic issues. No matter what your situation, the important thing is that you understand what is happening. Only then can you make informed decisions about how to move forward. And sometimes moving forward means stopping altogether.

In this chapter, we will talk about solving problems. We'll explore common recommendations, like when to use a nipple shield, triple feeding to support a low supply, how to handle gas and colic, and avoiding bottles to prevent nipple aversion. I will explain what a supplemental nursing system is and whether it makes sense for you. We'll also discuss pros and cons of craniosacral therapy and interventions for tongue tie and gape restriction, as well as what to expect afterward.

Nipple Shields

A nipple shield is a thin silicone covering that you put over your nipple and areola before nursing. It has openings over your nipple so your milk can come out. Nipple shields have been used for centuries, made from materials like pewter, silver, and animal skins. Rubber and latex varieties have also been tried more recently. The goal of nipple shields is to create a barrier between your baby's mouth and your nipples. They are routinely doled out by lactation consultants and labor and delivery nurses when they see moms struggling in the hospital or early postpartum period.

Before discussing appropriate use, let's consider why you would need a nipple shield in the first place. There are two main reasons: (1) to give your baby something to latch on to when he can't latch on to you and (2) because it hurts too much when you breastfeed. Both of those reasons, as you know now, are because your baby probably has a restricted gape, tongue tie, or both. We also know that if you don't fix the underlying problem, or at least acknowledge it, you'll keep running into trouble.

Since nipple pain and sliding off the breast come from a shallow latch, slapping on a nipple shield isn't going to fix anything. Although a nipple shield may give your baby something to put his mouth on, it doesn't change his gape or give him the ability to pull out milk. He will be able to take only what your breast gives him. In fact, if you try to nurse a baby with a normal gape using a nipple shield, he will have a harder time transferring milk. Nipple shields disrupt your baby's normal suck-and-swallow mechanisms. Unless you have a huge supply, your baby with a shallow latch won't get much milk with a shield. If you don't also pump to empty your breasts, you can eventually lose your supply, unless engorgement, plugged ducts, or mastitis get you first.

Something else happens when you use a nipple shield in the first few weeks. Because your baby's mouth can't directly stimulate your areola, the hormones responsible for laying down your supply can be disrupted. Of course, less stimulation is better than pain, but combined with reduced breast emptying, it can become more of a problem than a solution. It masks it only for a while. Except in certain circumstances, nipple shields aren't a fix. They are a Band-Aid that can get you only so far.

If your baby can't latch and has poor weight gain or you have pain, look for underlying problems. Check for a high palate and recessed chin. Look for tongue tie and a blister on his upper lip. Check for low tone. If your baby has a restricted gape and you have a huge supply, you can use a nipple shield, but know that you still have to pump out the rest of your milk. With or without the shield, if he has a shallow latch, your baby still won't get the fatty hindmilk, and eventually your breasts may stop producing. It may make more sense to just pump and bottle-feed to support your supply, unless you want your baby to undergo an intervention (see section below).

There are two ways nipple shields can actually be helpful, but both are in the context of first correcting a shallow latch with an intervention. If you have significant nipple damage, you can use a nipple shield as a barrier to help you heal, as you can continue nursing with his more normal latch. Also, if your baby has nipple aversion, you can use a nipple shield to transition him off the bottle and onto the breast. Keep in mind, however, that if you have already been using nipple shields, you may need to keep using them even after you correct his gape until you teach him through repeated feedings that he can nurse without them.

Triple Feeding

Triple feeding is a recommendation made by lactation consultants when your baby isn't gaining weight, usually for things like chronic cluster feeding, falling asleep at the breast, or any behavior that means your baby isn't transferring milk well. Moms are told to nurse for at least ten minutes on each side, then pump on each side and feed the baby that pumped milk. The process can add hours to your feeding time. Some moms spend the whole day doing it. The idea behind it is that continuing to nurse when your baby isn't getting milk from you will prevent him from forgetting your breast. We know that doesn't happen. If you think about this advice in the context of what you've learned, you can see how triple feeding on its own *creates* nipple confusion.

Triple feeding isn't always a cruel joke. It can be a way for you to check if your baby is better at transferring milk after he has an intervention for gape restriction or tongue tie. After your baby's latch is corrected, you should follow ten minutes of nursing with a short five-minute pump. You should have less milk to pump out and more in your baby. Pumping after nursing also pulls out any residual milk to help promote your supply. Triple feeding can help you get back on track after frenulectomies if your supply has dipped, but it is not meant as a long-term solution. I usually recommend a week at most.

Treating Nipple Aversion and the Myth of the Pacifier

Nipple aversion is often called *nipple confusion,* but it's more confusing for you than it is for your baby. As we already discussed, nipple aversion is a behavior babies learn when they are repeatedly made to breastfeed but can't get milk from the breast. This happens with either low supply or poor transfer as a result of a shallow latch or both. Once your baby learns he can't get milk from you, when you feed him with another source (because he will starve if you don't), he can quickly develop nipple aversion. He is not confused at all; he learns that the breast is the problem.

The best treatment for nipple aversion is to avoid it altogether. But that means going against common advice. If you have any of the symptoms of shallow latch, stop nursing and pump until you can address the underlying problem. Like I keep saying, your baby won't forget your breasts. If you stop nursing and pump for a few weeks, it's much easier to train him back onto your breasts than it is to overcome a negative association. His reflexes will stay intact unless you challenge them.

Giving him another food source, whether it is a bottle, cup, or syringe, won't prevent nipple aversion on its own. Moms are told to avoid bottles at all costs because they cause nipple aversion. Even the WHO "Ten Steps" protocol recommends against bottle use. But bottles themselves aren't the problem. If your baby is able to nurse from you, he will always prefer you.

The same is true for pacifiers. If your baby can breastfeed, there is no harm in giving him a pacifier. Studies have proven this.[1] In fact, studies have also shown that pacifier use encourages sucking and promotes breastfeeding and that restricting pacifier use decreases it.[2] Your baby can't get milk from a pacifier, so he will never choose it over your breast. Sucking on a pacifier helps soothe babies, but sucking on your breasts when he isn't getting milk isn't good for breastfeeding in the long run.

Once your baby has nipple aversion, there is no one-size-fits-all solution. You have to first address the latch or supply problem before you try to get them back on the breast. Here are some tricks to getting your baby back on the breast *after* you fix underlying gape restriction.

- **THE SOMBRERO:** Use a nipple shield for the first week so he starts to associate your breasts with milk. The plastic shield tricks him into thinking your breast is a bottle.
- **THE BAIT AND SWITCH:** Hold your baby in the cross-cradle position (see pages 26 and 60) using a nursing pillow. Get your breast ready to nurse by priming it. Feed your baby some milk from a bottle. Once he is calm, pull out the bottle and quickly switch it with your breast. You may need more than one set of hands to do this. Keep repeating until he sucks at your breast instead of crying for the bottle.
- **THE REBIRTH:** Get naked with your baby in a warm bath. Lay him on your chest and let him crawl to your breast, like you're mimicking the moment he was born. This works better with younger babies.

Dealing with an angry baby who refuses your breasts and goes crazy at the sight of them is no cakewalk. It's hard not to take it personally. Rejection is rejection, even if you understand why. Working with a patient lactation consultant can be very helpful. Helping your baby overcome nipple aversion takes patience, repetition, and a lot of crying (for both of you).

Supplemental Nursing System

A supplemental nursing system (SNS) is a very thin, soft silicone feeding tube that you tape to your breast with the opening at the nipple. The tube is attached to a bottle full of breastmilk or formula that is held above your breast to let the milk come out. The idea behind it is that it your baby can get milk from the tube when he can't get it from you. Besides being a clunky system, the motivation behind it is similar to that of a nipple shield. It is a Band-Aid that masks a problem rather than fixing it.

If your baby can't latch on to you and transfer milk, strapping on an outside source doesn't help him latch better. It just makes him less angry at your breasts. It also doesn't do anything to empty your breasts, so you have to pump. Common advice (that is thankfully waning) is for moms to nurse, pump, then feed with an SNS. It is believed that keeping your baby at your breast, even if he isn't transferring milk, will prevent nipple aversion. But if you take a step back, you can see how this makes no sense. If your baby can't transfer out your milk, an SNS is just theatrics. It's not only a waste of time, but poor transfer is usually the result of a painful, shallow latch, which can also reduce your supply. An SNS should never be used if you have a huge supply.

SNS can be helpful, but only when you have a low supply and your baby has a normal latch. If your baby has a shallow latch, you must first correct it. Once you know your baby is able to transfer milk, you can use an SNS as a positive reinforcement to get him back on your breast. The SNS provides extra milk or formula to keep him nursing so he associates your breast with food. When you have a low supply, you can use this method as long as you like. If you find it cumbersome, you can always nurse for five to ten minutes on each breast, so your baby gets out what you have, then switch to a bottle.

Craniosacral Therapy

Over the past twenty years, the use of osteopathy for babies has grown. Osteopathy is a kind of medicine based on the idea that form determines function. Using physical contact, the body can self-heal structural imbalances. Unlike chiropractics or massage, there is no rubbing, pushing, or cracking. The touch is very gentle, and sometimes it is barely felt at all.

Cranial osteopathy is a very specialized treatment performed by doctors of osteopathy (DOs). Craniosacral therapy (CST) is a watered-down version that anyone can perform, but is usually done by physical therapists. The difference in cost is quite large. Make sure you check credentials before you let anyone touch your baby. Although it is best to see a DO, there are talented craniosacral therapists who specialize in newborns. Ideally, your baby can be treated shortly after he's born for a single visit or a series of four treatments.

The reason to seek CST is for gentle repositioning to balance asymmetries from womb position or delivery type. For example, CST can release the nerves at the base of the skull that may have been compressed during a vaginal birth. It can release tension in jaw muscles and allow the *vagus nerve,* a cranial nerve that affects the gut, to calm down and reduce reflux. CST also supports waking up a sleepy baby's reflexes and helping babies with suck disorder. CST is safe for all infants, in the right hands. In many cases, gentle repositioning can support frenulectomies when babies have severe gape restriction. CST alone can't correct gape restriction.

Treating Gas and Colic: Holds, Feeding, Bottle Nipples

Now that you understand what causes gas and colic, fixing it seems pretty straightforward. You can do an elimination diet to see if your diet is the culprit. You can also treat your baby's underlying gape restriction and high palate with frenulectomies. Few bottle nipples on the market help with gas, even though most of them promise to. One nipple, called the *Haberman feeder,* was designed for babies with cleft palate, to fill the open space in the palate. It can also help fill a high palate.

There are certain holds that help your baby move out extra gas. Babies cry from gas because it hurts when their stomach and intestines get stretched out. They try to move out the gas by arching their backs, kicking, and grunting. But you can help your baby by decompressing his belly with your hands. Here are some holds that help relieve gas distention. Bouncing your baby gently while you do the holds also helps.

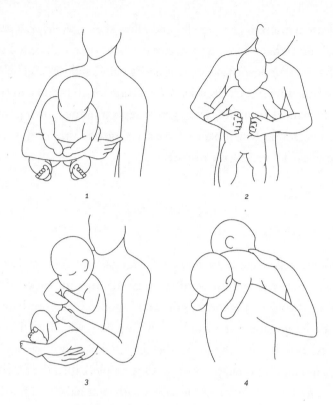

1. Hold your baby and place your left arm around his belly. Lean him forward, allowing his weight against your arm to compress the gas out.

2. Using both hands, grasp your baby with your fingers on his belly. Squeeze gently while bouncing him in a seated position on your knee or a table.

3. Using one arm under your baby's legs, bend him into a seated position, using that arm as a chair. Curve the fingers of your other hand and press them into the soft part of his belly, leaning him forward as you do it. Bounce him this way to move the air out.

4. Hold your baby over your shoulder, with your shoulder in the soft part of his belly.

Home remedies that calm your baby's gas and colic are chamomile tea and gripe water. If your baby is one month or older, you can buy gripe water or make your own by boiling one teaspoon of fennel in one cup of water for ten minutes. Cool, then give your baby a few drops throughout the day with a dropper. Gas drops that contain simethicone, which breaks up air bubbles, are also safe for babies. Avoid drops with benzoic acid or sodium benzoate, which are unsafe in large amounts.

If you've tried everything and nothing works, you may want to speak to your pediatrician about medication. I think reflux medication is overused in babies, but there are times when it is the only thing that works. Preparations of reflux medications for newborns are usually made in a compounding pharmacy in a liquid form. Work with your pediatrician before starting any medication.

Because babies with a high palate, gape restriction, and tongue tie swallow a lot of air, treating your baby with frenulectomies will also resolve their gas and colic. This helps whether your baby is breastfed, bottle-fed, or both.

Surgery

Treating gape restriction and tongue tie has become popular over the past ten years. When you look at the skyrocketing number of procedures being performed, you may wonder whether we are witnessing an epidemic of tethered tongues or if these things are being overdiagnosed. It's actually a little bit of both. In the past, moms figured out how to feed their babies using whatever worked. But even today, in places where breast-feeding is the only option, only 60 percent of babies are able to do it past six months. Nowadays, moms want to breastfeed their babies on their own breasts. It's not that gape restriction and tongue tie are any more prevalent now than they were in the past. The difference is that now there is a treatment that works. Most of the time.

Frenulectomy, frenulotomy, and frenotomy are different words describe the removal or division of a frenulum. A frenulum is just connective tissue that holds two structures together. In your baby's mouth, we are primarily talking about the frenulum under his upper lip and the one under his tongue.

If your baby's tongue is more than 75 percent tied, I recommend he have a frenulectomy as soon as possible. Early treatment with this procedure can be done in an office, has little chance of growing back, and has an easy recovery. The tongue is a muscle, so the earlier you release it, the easier it is for the tongue to develop normally on its own. There is no reason to wait, because, contrary to popular opinion, tongue ties never stretch out or go away on their own.

Most babies with tongue tie will also have trouble nursing. Studies have shown that performing frenulectomies increases milk transfer, decreases nipple pain, and helps babies stay latched on. But tongue tie is often missed by pediatricians. If you suspect a tongue tie, you can easily check for yourself by placing your pointer and middle finger under your baby's tongue and lifting up. If he has tongue tie, you will see a band of tissue near the tip of his tongue. Treating an obvious tongue tie early will save you and your baby a lot of trouble later on.

Using frenulectomies in any other circumstance is controversial. As I explained in Chapter 10, there is no such thing as a posterior tongue tie or lip tie, but lip and tongue frenulectomies are excellent treatments for gape restriction. The caveat is that both have to be done at the same time, regardless of whether your baby also has tongue tie. Releasing both frenula allows your baby's palate, tongue, and jaw to move independently from one another so he can unhinge his jaw to gape and latch on deeply. Gape restriction matters only for the first year of feeding.

When you take your baby in for frenulectomies, you are often made to believe the procedures will fix breastfeeding, but that simply isn't true. If done correctly, frenulectomies are 100 percent effective in releasing gape restriction, but that is all they do. But there are a lot of variables involved in breastfeeding, and you have to take them all into account. For example, if you have a low supply and your baby is refusing the breast, after you release his gape, you still have to deal with low supply and nipple aversion. On the other hand, if you have a good supply and your baby is very young, the chances are much better that releasing his gape will be enough to save nursing. Every situation has to be considered individually.

But simply performing the procedure doesn't automatically fix breastfeeding. After your baby's gape is released, he still has to *fit* enough of your breast into his mouth to fill his high palate. Just latching him on and letting go may not be enough. This is where frenulectomies get blamed for not working. Just because your baby's gape is released, it doesn't mean your breast will automatically fit the shape of the inside of his mouth. You should check your baby's gape and latch before you leave the office by using the cross-cradle hold (see Chapter 4). Your baby's gape should immediately be noticeably wider and unhinged, allowing for a much deeper latch. Most of your areola should be inside your baby's mouth, and he should form a seal with his upper lip flanged out. His swallowing will be deeper, which you can see by looking under his jaw. You can also feel that he can pull out more milk.

Frenulectomies are even more controversial when it comes to deciding which babies should undergo the procedures. If your baby is diagnosed with "lip tie" or "posterior tongue tie," be wary. The only reason to do procedures on these babies is to release the gape. Period. They won't have any of the issues tongue-tied babies have because they don't actually have tongue tie. Even so, it's hard to guess ahead of time who will benefit from the procedures. Tongue ties occur in 4 to 10 percent of the population, but around 20 percent of babies have trouble nursing. Most breastfeeding struggles happen from gape restriction, but there may also be a tongue tie. You have to check for both. There is also no accepted protocol for how the procedures should be done and who should be doing them. There is no formalized training program—doctors and dentists figure it out on their own. Make sure you ask the right questions (page 181–82) before going forward with the procedure.

Patient Perspective

Baby Lila, almost six months old, has had trouble nursing since she was born. She had a frenulectomy to release her tongue frenulum when she was two months old. Her nursing got better, and she was able to nurse for a longer time at each session. But her nursing problems crept up, gradually becoming worse. The baby nursed for a short period of time and transferred very little milk. Mom's supply was still good, but that was only because she had been pumping and taking supplements to boost her supply. She took Lila to a new pediatrician who is also an IBCLC, who referred them to me. Mom is still breastfeeding, with plans to continue, but would like some guidance.

On exam, Lila had a high, wide palate with only minimal regrowth of Type 1 tongue tie. She had restricted gape because of her high palate, and she was easily distressed by the breast.

I discussed a re-excision with her mom at length. Because the baby already has breast aversion and was nearly six months old, doing another procedure may have widened her gape, but ultimately would not have improved the quality of breastfeeding. Her mom deferred the procedure and continued pumping and bottle-feeding. Because the baby's tongue movement would not inhibit eating in the future, no procedure was warranted.

For some mom-and-baby dyads, even after the procedure, the baby still doesn't fit onto the breast. Usually this is because the baby has a very high, cupped palate. You can try adding craniosacral therapy, but many moms are pushed to do more invasive procedures. I caution you against this, unless you get more than one opinion. The procedure is only the first step. The *goal* is successful breastfeeding. But it doesn't work for everyone. While no one has done studies on this, the effect of frenulectomies on breastfeeding in my practice is as follows:

- 65 to 70 percent are like magic and fix breastfeeding right away.
- 20 to 25 percent see improvement in symptoms, but other help is needed.
- 5 to 10 percent don't help at all.

These procedures are not the panacea they are made out to be. They can help, but you may still need other support, like seeing a lactation consultant and craniosacral therapy. You also need time and patience. If this all feels like too much, you may decide to pump and bottle-feed, or bottle-feed with formula—and that's okay too.

14

Going Back to Work

Regardless of when you have to return to work, it will be a big change from what you're used to. For some moms, going back to work means working from home. But for most, it means returning to the office and leaving your baby with another caregiver. Whether it's a nanny, a close relative, or daycare, handing your baby off to someone else can be one of the hardest things you do, especially because you've been such a vital part of her existence.

I can relate. Leaving my baby when I had to go back to my residency program after only six weeks felt like I was losing a limb. After I gave birth, the way I navigated the world had completely changed. I missed her so much, I used to go to the pediatric ICU at the hospital and sit with the sick babies. During the first pediatric tracheotomy I performed, I broke down in tears. Every time I scrubbed in to a case, I worried I would leak through my surgical scrubs. There was nowhere to pump because male and female residents shared the same call room. By the time I got home, my daughter was already asleep, but I stayed up and held her despite my sleep deprivation. It was one of the hardest times of my life.

Going back to work can feel like a loss, but it doesn't have to. It also doesn't mean you have to stop breastfeeding. Breastfeeding can be an important way stay connected to your baby. The bond you've already established through healthy breastfeeding, no matter what that looks like, can fill the void of missing your baby. It won't be easy, but I have some suggestions to make your transition less stressful. A lot of it boils down to attitude. If you feel embarrassed or shy about pumping at work, think about how much you love your baby. When you set limits for meetings so you can pump, feel proud of yourself instead of worrying how others see you. If you're relieved to get time away from your baby, don't feel guilty about it.

In this chapter we will look at how your breastfeeding relationship changes as you transition back to work. The end of your maternity leave brings a lot of mixed emotions. We will discuss the where, how, and when to pump at work to keep your supply going, tips on maintaining your supply, and how to make the whole thing easier on yourself. I will give you tools so you can advocate for yourself in the workplace and at home, making sure you have the support you need from your partner, family, and other caregivers. But first, we need to acknowledge the importance of self-care.

Self-Care

Getting and maintaining balance can be hard as you transition. You may be sad that you are giving too much some days and guilty that you aren't giving enough on others. But, as they say on the airplane, you have to put on your own mask first. You have to take care of yourself if you want to keep going, and that doesn't make you selfish. It is easy to throw yourself into work and then give everything you have to your baby and your family when you get home. Don't do it. Each day, no matter how busy you are, take at least ten minutes for yourself.

These ten minutes can be as simple as sitting in silence or meditating. Stretching is also good to get your blood flowing. Energy can get trapped in your muscles if you don't move and stretch. Going for a quick walk by yourself helps. Writing. Anything is fine as long as you do it alone. It may not be easy, and everyone around you may beg for your attention. But this time is vital, even if you have to fight for it. Ask your partner or nanny for help. Establish a routine early, and pretty soon it will feel natural.

Another part of self-care is diet. As you rush to leave the house, don't just grab whatever's easiest. Plan your meals, prepare them ahead of time, hire a food delivery service, take your prenatal vitamins and extra vitamin D. Make sure you are eating balanced meals and avoiding excess sugar and processed foods.

As corny as this sounds, forgive yourself for leaving your baby. Know you are making the right choices, which also includes taking care of your needs. Many moms don't have a choice about returning to work. Some are the primary breadwinner or the only one. Giving birth and nursing while trying to earn a living is a heavy load to carry. Even if working is a choice, know that you can have it all but not at the same time. Your baby won't be a baby forever. Her needs will change as she gets older, but your needs are important too. You deserve help. You are still a mom even if you don't do everything yourself. Give yourself time to adjust to your changing role.

Benefits of Breastfeeding when You Return to Work

Although some moms want to throw in the towel when they go back to work, there are benefits to continuing to breastfeed. Once your bond is established, breastfeeding is wonderful way to sustain it. It can help you stay connected even though you aren't spending as much time at home. That oxytocin can be good for you and your baby at the end of the workday.

There are also the benefits of breastmilk itself, including antibodies and customized nutrition. Pumped milk is just as good as milk taken directly from the breast. Even if you can't provide everything your baby needs, any amount of breastmilk helps.

Preparing to Go Back to Work

Often, the difference between success and extra stress is preparation. As your return-to-work date approaches, start to transition to your new schedule slowly. Establish a pumping routine beginning in the second or third week. You should learn how your pump works and how you react to your pump. Not everyone can pump effectively with the machine alone. Some moms need hand stimulation and/or their baby to get oxytocin going and initiate a letdown.

Pumping can also allow other caregivers to help you with feedings. Your baby may not take a bottle from you, preferring your breasts when she smells you. Let other people feed your baby so she doesn't refuse the bottle when it's time for you to leave.

While pumping, you can also start building some milk stores. You don't need a freezer full of milk, so don't make yourself crazy. Having a few days' worth of milk at a time is usually enough of a buffer, especially because you will be pumping at work and nursing when you are home. As we know from Chapter 8, babies need 28 to 32 ounces a day from one month until you stop nursing. Smaller babies will take less at a time and eat more often than older babies. During a typical eight-hour workday, plan to have 12 to 24 ounces per day, for a total of 36 to 72 ounces stored at a time. You can collect the extra milk this way:

- Pump three times a day, after you nurse, to get what's left behind.
- Pump at the same time each day.
- Make the first pump after your first feed, because mornings are when you make the most milk.
- Pump for only eight to ten minutes per session.
- Massage your breasts or do hand stimulation before you pump.

Store milk as recommended (see Chapter 8), and try to use it within six months of pumping.

Choosing a Caregiver

You may be lucky enough to have a family member or trusted nanny to care for your baby. Or you may need to find a daycare or friend to help out. Whoever you choose, the caregiver should understand your breastfeeding goals and support them. Not all childcare providers know how to handle breastmilk safely, especially if they are caring for more than one child. Have this conversation beforehand, including any individual instructions. Your provider should be happy to feed your baby your pumped milk and have a safe place to store it. Make sure you leave them with enough sanitized bottles and that they understand how to warm breastmilk. In some situations, you may want to find a provider near your job so you can visit your baby on your lunch break to nurse her. You may also want to nurse her right away when you pick her up.

Know Your Rights

What you may not realize is that you have the right to breastfeed at work. The Patient Protection and Affordable Care Act requires nearly all employers to offer you reasonable break times to pump for up to a year after your baby is born. And I don't mean a bathroom or public area. They have to give you a private, comfortable, safe place to pump and time to do it.

It helps to have conversations with your employer before

you go back to work. They may not have experience with nursing moms, and you need them to be on your side when you start back. The website Supporting Nursing Moms at Work: Employer Solutions (www.womenshealth.gov/supporting-nursing-moms-work) has a lot of tips and solutions. It can help your employer help you, regardless of your type of workplace. Discuss how you will need to adjust your schedule, even if it means working part-time or splitting shifts. You should budget time during the day for pumping. Learn about the Break Time for Nursing Mothers federal law that also protects your nursing and pumping time.

Pumping Advice

You need a good strategy for pumping before you go back to work. The last thing you need is to be trapped in a meeting with bursting breasts with nowhere to relieve them. If there are other moms who currently are or have pumped at your workplace, ask them for advice and support. They can help you problem-solve and avoid pitfalls they may have suffered.

When it comes to pumping, there are a number of things to consider:

- *Where to pump:* You need privacy, a calm environment, a comfortable chair, a sink to wash your pumping supplies, and an electrical outlet. If it's big or progressive enough, your workplace may have a lactation lounge, or you can convince them to create one. A corporate lactation program could include a delegated room, hospital-grade pumps, and a place to store milk. Check the schedule so you don't overlap with other pumping moms. You can always pump at your desk if you have a private office, and hang a Do Not Disturb sign on the door. If you work in a hospital, maternity wards often have pumping rooms. It may be challenging to find appropriate space in other worksites, but under no circumstances is a bathroom an acceptable option.

- *When to pump:* It is best to pump as often as your baby nurses. Smaller babies nurse every two to three hours, and older babies every four to six hours. If you work eight hours a day, that means three pumps: midmorning, lunchtime, and midafternoon, with the possibility of decreasing to twice a day as time goes on. You need to empty your breasts to keep them filling up, but you also need to pump enough so you don't end up with plugged ducts or mastitis. I strongly suggest pumping both breasts at the same time for about fifteen minutes. Depending on your job, you may have to go in earlier or stay later to make up for the time you spend pumping. You may also want to schedule pumping sessions into your calendar so you aren't disturbed. Put reminders on your phone. Let your coworkers know your pumping schedule. Place a hard stop on meeting times. And no matter how busy you get, stay on schedule as much as you can.

- *How to pump:* While it is tempting to continue working while you pump, it's a better idea to relax, look at pictures of your baby, and shift gears into a calmer state of mind. Bringing something to work that smells like your baby also helps. Anything to get that oxytocin going will help your letdown kick in and your breasts empty more completely.

- *Where to store milk:* Bring your own cooler with ice packs or an insulated bag you can store in a fridge at work. Make sure to clearly mark your bottles or bags of milk. Remember these storage guidelines for breastmilk:

  - Room temperature for 6 to 8 hours
  - Insulated cooler bag with ice packs for 24 hours
  - Fridge for 5 days
  - Freezer for 3 to 6 months
  - Deep freeze for 6 to 12 months

- *How to dress:* Nursing tops and bras are really helpful, but you may have a different dress code at work, so a good option is something with buttons or a zipper in front. That way you don't have to totally disrobe to pump. It's also a good idea to keep an extra set of tops, jackets, and bras and lots of extra breast pads in case you leak.

- *What to bring:* You may want to keep a pump at work and one at home. If that's cost-prohibitive for you, then you'll have to carry it back and forth. You can save cleaning time by storing your pump parts in the fridge during the day. You can also get two sets of attachments, one for each location. If your workplace has pumps, just buy the attachments and leave them at work. Bring extra pump bags and bottles for storage, a freezer bag, and a cooler. Some moms carry around a hand pump in case of emergencies.

When You Get Home

No matter how long you're at work, it may seem like a long time to be away from your baby. When you do see her again, take time to reconnect. This may be simply holding and playing with her. It could also be bathing or nursing her. You don't have to nurse all the time when you are home, but it can be a good way to reconnect. Your baby may want to nurse more often at night, when you are home, and eat less during the day. This is called *reverse-cycling*. If your baby gets a lot from you overnight, you may not need to store as much milk during the day, but keep your breasts emptied so you don't lose your supply.

Don't feel bad about asking for help, even when you're home. Your partner can still bottle-feed while you rest or take time for yourself. You don't have to be on all the time to be a good mom. And it's good for your baby to have a community of caregivers. It takes a village, for your baby and you.

15

Thanks for the Mammaries

Although, as moms, we may feel like we are emotionally breastfeeding our entire lives, the physical act of doing it usually is much shorter. You may nurse for two months or continue for several years. Every mom, baby, and situation is different. Hopefully you've had a wonderful experience and learned a lot along the way. You have given your heart and soul and body to this venture, and you should feel proud regardless of how long it lasted. Now that you've come to the end of your breastfeeding journey, congratulations on a job well done! It's time to wean.

Weaning is defined as the act or process of causing a baby to stop feeding on its mother's milk and start eating other food, including formula. The key word is *causing*. This implies a conscious choice. But not everything we call weaning is a choice. Weaning is a natural part of breastfeeding and starts even when nursing is going well, when you give your baby solid food at age six months. It can also happen earlier for personal reasons. But in many cases, breastfeeding ends even though you don't want it to. For example, your baby may have low tone, or you may get sick. Why you stop nursing is mostly the result of medical, physiological, and anatomical reasons that are beyond your control. A breastfeeding relationship that falls apart when you want to keep going is very different from one based on a conscious decision to stop. Breastfeeding failure is not the same as weaning. Failure is not a choice.

In this chapter, we will differentiate between weaning circumstances that are beyond your control and those that are your choice. We will also talk about how and when to start weaning, based on your baby's age and your life circumstances. Finally, I will also discuss how to take care of yourself during and after the process.

Types of Weaning

I hesitate to classify weaning into the usual groups, like baby-led, gradual, and sudden, because failure is grouped together with other kinds of weaning. They are not the same thing. Your baby may stop nursing because he isn't transferring milk. You can call this baby-led, but that discounts the underlying reason. You may stop nursing because your supply runs out, but that's not the same as choosing to decrease your supply. There is a big difference, emotionally and physically, between wanting to stop and having to stop. Nursing cessation is more accurately divided into two groups:

- *Not your decision:* These reasons to stop breastfeeding aren't simply a choice. They usually involve underlying medical, anatomical, and physiological conditions that either end breastfeeding on their own or force you to stop, even if you don't want to.

- Baby stops on his own (sudden or gradual) because of poor transfer from a shallow latch, low supply, change in milk flavor, or reasons no one can figure out.
- Your breasts stop making milk because of inherently low supply, poor transfer from a shallow latch, pregnancy, or other hormonal changes.
- You have to take medication that's unsafe for your baby because of infection, medical problems like depression and hypothyroidism, cancer, accidents, or emergency.
- You are having trouble getting pregnant again so you are going through fertility treatments.
- You get your period, which changes the flavor of your milk and can reduce your supply.
- Your baby can't digest milk protein, which is a metabolic problem requiring special formula.
- You get sick and need surgery or hospitalization because of cancer, accident, infection, and so on.

- *Your decision:* These are examples of situations when you could continue but you decide to stop.

  - You make very little milk (because of inherently low supply or loss of supply from a shallow latch, not emptying your breasts often, etc.), so you figure, why bother?

- You have terrible pain from a shallow latch, Raynaud's, poor fit, or all of the above, despite frenulectomies.
- You have to go back to work and you can't or don't want to pump. Your job may not make it possible, you don't have time, or maybe you travel often.
- You want your life and your body back so you can eat and drink whatever you want and have your own schedule.
- You get pregnant again and don't want to keep nursing.
- You, or others around you, think your baby is too old. It should be your decision, but peer pressure is real.
- Your baby gets teeth and it scares you. Teeth shouldn't mean an end to nursing, but it's your choice.
- Your baby starts kindergarten or elementary school. Just kidding. Sort of.

When to Start Weaning

Regardless of the reason, there is always guilt when you stop nursing. Seeing your baby's wide-open mouth and huge, hungry eyes, knowing he's not going to get your breast, is heartbreaking. It's even worse if you are being made to stop and you don't want to. Just know this is only the first of many times you have to say no to your baby. It may not get any easier, but rest assured, a huge part of good parenting is disappointing your child.

The recommended goal for exclusive breastfeeding by the WHO and the American Academy of Pediatrics is for the first six months. This is a great benchmark, but it's not possible or desirable for everyone. Nursing your baby less than six months doesn't hurt him. There is no maximum time you can breast-feed, either, although society has its own opinions. There is no shame in nursing a toddler. As long as you aren't forced to stop, you get to decide how long is long enough.

Most babies decide they are done nursing between nine and twelve months, but some go on for longer. If your baby decides to stop early, it is likely because of a sudden drop in your sup-ply or a change in its taste, which happens when you get your period. Most of the time, we have no idea why babies stop nursing.

When you decide to wean, you have to consider the two parts of breastfeeding: your supply and your baby's attachment to nursing from you. If you have a major life change, like mov-ing or going back to work, it's best to wean slowly so you and your baby can ease through the transition. Try to avoid wean-ing when he is teething or sick, so he can have you to comfort him through the rough patches. You may start to wean and then change your mind, or decide to partially wean so he just nurses a few times a day. All babies are different and have their own way of tolerating weaning. It can be an easy transition or a stressful one.

You may have a plentiful supply but are forced to stop because of a medical reason. If your baby has a milk allergy, for instance, you won't be able to feed him your milk. Consider donating to a milk bank as you slow down your supply. You may have a medical condition that requires you to take medication that isn't compatible with nursing. If so, you have to pump and dump until you stop lactating. If you have a medical condition that suddenly stops your milk production, at least you don't have to slow your supply. Some moms get sick and have to take a medication, like steroids, that stops their supply. Others are diagnosed with life-threatening illnesses or need surgery, so their nursing is the last thing on their minds. Every condition is unique, and you should work with your OB/GYN and/or lactation consultant when slowing or stopping your supply for medical reasons. No matter the reason, stopping an abundant supply always sucks.

How to Wean

You have to wean based on your supply and your baby's age. Sometimes weaning is easier when your baby is younger than three months because he isn't as attached as an older baby. The key is to go slowly, giving him and your breasts the time they need.

- *0 to 6 months:* Wean by substituting bottles for nursing sessions. Start a few weeks ahead of your weaning date or before your baby is six weeks old by adding in one or two bottles a day. If you wait until he is three or four months old to introduce bottles, he may refuse them.

The bottles can contain breastmilk or formula. Drop one feeding every three to four days so weaning can be complete by two weeks. You can give him the bottles, or you can have someone else do it if he won't take them from you.

You have to also pump just enough to prevent your breasts from being uncomfortable, but not enough to empty them. Usually this takes three minutes or less. Do the opposite of what keeps your breasts producing milk. If you are weaning during the first few months, you should slowly taper down your nursing and pumping to prevent engorgement, plugged ducts, and mastitis. Your milk supply may take longer to wean than it takes to stop your baby nursing from your breast, but you can always feed him that milk in a bottle. If your supply is unmanageable, you can work with a doctor or lactation consultant and take supplements or medications to stop milk production (see Chapter 11).

- *6 to 12 months:* At six months, you can wean your baby with a bottle or go directly to a sippy cup. Choose a spill-proof cup with a spout. Remember that your baby needs breastmilk or formula for the first year, so you should gradually replace one nursing session a day with a bottle or cup. It's easiest to replace early-morning or daytime feedings first.

Bedtime nursing is usually the last to go. Around nine months, babies often lose interest in nursing on their own. No one knows why, but it may be partly because of their growing interest in the outside world. However, that same age group can also suffer from separation anxiety and get clingier than ever. You can exchange nursing with extra attention and a lot of skin-to-skin contact. Snuggling or reading together can replace the oxytocin you will both miss from breastfeeding. You can also use distraction when he is pining for the breast by using play or make-believe.

At six months you can start introducing solids. Iron-fortified rice cereal is usually recommended first, because it is hypoallergenic. Speaking of allergies, if you have a history of them or your baby reacted to certain foods through your breastmilk, keep a diary of what you feed him. Add strained fruits and vegetables one at a time, waiting a few days in between to see if he reacts.

At first, you can try blended fruits and vegetables that aren't too sweet. You should also avoid added salt, which can overload his kidneys. Broccoli, sweet potatoes, carrots, apples, or pears are a good start. You can also try peas, squash, eggplant, spinach, green beans, and cauliflower. Later, you can add bananas, mashed berries, pineapple, mango, peaches, and plums. After seven months, you can offer your baby pureed meats, ground table food, and finger foods. Avoid nuts, grapes, or anything small enough to cause choking. As your baby gets older, you can try different textures and finger foods, or give him a spoon so he can try to feed himself. Whole cow's milk and honey is only safe after your baby turns one year old, so avoid them until then. Eggs and fish should be fully cooked.

Your supply may be easier to suppress after six months. Unless you are a big producer, slowly tapering off nursing by dropping a session a day and replacing it with a bottle of pumped milk or formula can get your baby weaned within two weeks. If you have a huge supply and have to take it slower, that's fine. The later you wean, the faster your milk dries up, so plan for that possibility. Chapter 11 has a list of supplements, medications, and foods that can quickly stop milk production.

- *Over a year:* After a year, your baby can drink cow's milk or other fortified milk substitutes. You can wean directly onto a sippy cup because all babies should be off the bottle by one year. Because of all the time you've spent together, it is sometimes harder to wean a toddler than it is a younger baby. You may be able to wean most of the daytime feeds and be left with bedtime nursing, especially if you co-sleep. Putting him in his own bed can help, but you will have to battle that separately. Try dropping a session every few days, shortening each session, and increasing the time between feeds. The more active he is, the less he will notice a skipped session. Conversely, some toddlers just wake up one day and want to stop.

Partial Weaning

If your supply has waned or you want to limit nursing, you can wean down to a few nursing sessions a day. Breastfeeding isn't all or none. You may want to nurse first thing in the morning and once in the evening, which works well if you're back to working a nine-to-five job. You may want to nurse only once a day and avoid pumping altogether. Some moms can sustain this for months and even years, depending on supply.

Post-Weaning Depression

Whether you decide to wean or it is thrust upon you, the process is always emotional. You may feel relieved that a hard situation is over but also feel sad for the loss. You may be happy that you have your life back but guilty for choosing yourself over your baby. Weaning is emotional and sometimes depressing. Your feelings aren't all based on what's actually happening. If you've had a good breastfeeding relationship, you lose oxytocin when you stop nursing. If your breastfeeding relationship has been rough, you have an increased risk of postpartum depression for up to six months after you stop nursing.

Hormonal shifts are real. They may make you feel like you're living in someone else's body. Your mood can shift from day to day, hour to hour, and there may be no rhyme or reason. Take it easy on yourself. This is the perfect time for meditation, yoga, alone time, anything that helps you find your center again. Don't try to handle these emotions alone. At the very least, talk to your partner, parents, friends, and support network. Your doula or lactation consultant can recommend support groups. Your doctor can refer you for specialized therapy or treatment.

Gratitude

I encourage all moms to do a ritual to close out their breastfeeding journey. It starts with giving thanks. For your baby. For the gift of motherhood. For the ability to feed your baby. No amount is too small. No time is too short. Whether your breastfeeding dreams came true or you were met with heartbreak, being grateful for what you were given can heal all wounds. You are changed now. No matter how you ended up feeding your baby, you are a mother. You created life.

ACKNOWLEDGMENTS

This book has been eighteen years in the making, even before I knew it had to be written. I will be forever grateful to my agent, Iris Blasi, and my editor, Michele Eniclerico, who took it on even though there were already too many breastfeeding books and my perspective was way outside the box. Without them and everyone at Rodale, it would still be knocking around in my head, fighting to get out. I want to thank my daughter, Lucy, for showing me the true definition of motherhood.

I owe a debt of gratitude to all the lactation consultants, nurse practitioners, midwives, doulas, osteopaths, and pediatricians I've worked with over the years, who taught me so much. There are far too many to mention. And to all mothers and fathers who trusted me with their babies.

A special thank-you to my loved ones, who've championed my efforts and taught me the true meaning of friendship. Jodi Stein and Charlie Alterman, my always companions, for reading everything I write and saying it's the best thing they've ever read even when it isn't. Dr. Yael Halaas, who predicted, when we first met, I would move to New York and become her best friend, and she was right. Diane Moore, for being the best sister in the world. Dr. Darius Kohan and Joe Agosta, two of the kindest, most generous human beings alive.

NOTES

CHAPTER 2

1. H. W. Korsmo, X. Jiang, and M. Caudill, "Choline: Exploring the Growing Science on Its Benefits for Moms and Babies," *Nutrients* 11, no. 8 (Aug. 2019): 1823. doi: 10.3390/nu11081823.

CHAPTER 3

1. M. Sanches, "Clinical Management of Oral Disorders in Breast-feeding," *Jorno de Pediatria* 80, suppl. no. 5 (Nov. 2004): S155–62. doi: 10.2223/1249.
2. F. Weber, M. Woolridge, and J. D. Baum, "Ultrasonographic Study of the Organisation of Sucking and Swallowing by Newborn Infants," *Developmental Medicine & Child Neurology* 28, no. 1 (Feb. 1986): 19–24. doi: 10.1111/j.1469-8749.1986.tb03825.
3. M. Sohn, Y. Ahn, and S. Lee, "Assessment of Primitive Reflexes in High-Risk Newborns," *Journal of Clinical Medical Research* 3, no. 6 (Dec. 2011): 285–90.
4. D. T. Geddes, L. Chadwick, J. Kent, C. Garbin, and P. Hartmann, "Ultrasound Imaging of Infant Swallowing During Breastfeeding," *Dysphagia* 25, no. 3 (Sept. 2010): 183–91. doi: 10.1007/s00455-009 -9241-0.
5. C. Watson and W. Khaled, "Mammary Development in the Embryo and Adult: A Journey of Morphogenesis and Commitment," *Development* 135, no. 6 (Mar. 2008): 995–1003. doi: 10.1242/dev .005439.

6. K. Uvnäs-Moberg, et al. "Maternal Plasma Levels of Oxytocin During Breastfeeding—A Systematic Review," *PLoS One* 15, no. 8 (2020): e0235806. doi: 10.1371/journal.pone.0235806.

7. H. Gardner, J. Kent, C. T. Lai, L. R. Mitoulas, M. D. Cregan, P. Hartmann, and D. Geddes, "Milk Ejection Patterns: An Intra-individual Comparison of Breastfeeding and Pumping," *BMC Pregnancy Childbirth* 15 (2015): 156. doi: 10.1186/s12884-015-0583-3.

8. D. K. Prime, D. Geddes, and P. E. Hartmann, "Oxytocin: Milk Ejection and Maternal-Infant Well-Being," in *Textbook of Human Lactation,* edited by T. W. Hale and P. E. Hartmann, vol. 1. Amarillo, Texas: Hale Publishing; 2007. p. 141–58.

9. M. Neville, T. McFadden, and I. Forsyth, "Hormonal Regulation of Mammary Differentiation and Milk Secretion," *Journal of Mammary Gland Biology and Neoplasia* 7, no. 1 (Jan. 2002): 49–66. doi: 10.1023/a:1015770423167.

10. D. B. Cox, R. A. Owens, and P. E. Hartmann, "Blood and Milk Prolactin and the Rate of Milk Synthesis in Women," *Experimental Physiology* 81, no. 6 (Nov. 1996): 1007–20.

11. M. Peaker and C. J. Wilde, "Feedback Control of Milk Secretion from Milk," *Journal of Mammary Gland Biology and Neoplasia* 1, no. 3 (July 1996): 307–15. doi: 10.1007/BF02018083.

CHAPTER 4

1. S. Doucet, R. Soussignan, P. Sagot, and B. Schaal, "The Secretion of Areolar (Montgomery's) Glands from Lactating Women Elicits Selective, Unconditional Responses in Neonates," *PLoS One* 4, no. 10 (2009): e7579. doi: 10.1371/journal.pone.0007579.

2. J. Morton, "Hand Expression of Breastmilk," Stanford Medicine / Newborn Nursery at Lucile Packard Children's Hospital. https://med.stanford.edu/newborns/professional-education/breastfeeding/hand-expressing-milk.html.

CHAPTER 5

1. B. Fischer and P. Mitteroecker, "Covariation Between Human Pelvis Shape, Stature, and Head Size Alleviates the Obstetric Dilemma," *Proceedings of the National Academy of Sciences of the United*

States of America 112, no. 18 (May 2015): 5655–60. doi: 10.1073
/pnas.1420325112.

2. R. Sunderland, "Fetal Position and Skull Shape," *British Journal of Obstetrics and Gynaecology* 88, no. 3 (Mar. 1981): 246–49. doi: 10.1111/j.1471-0528.1981.tb00976.

3. O. Ami, J. Maran, P. Gabor, E. Whitacre, D. Musset, C. Dubray, G. Mage, and L. Boyer, "Three-Dimensional Magnetic Resonance Imaging of Fetal Head Molding and Brain Shape Changes During the Second Stage of Labor," *PLoS One* 14, no. 5 (May 2019): e0215721. doi: 10.1371/journal.pone.0215721.

4. J. Allen, J. Parratt, M. Rolfe, C. Hastie, A. Saxton, K. Fahy, "Immediate, Uninterrupted Skin-to-Skin Contact and Breastfeeding After Birth: A Cross-Sectional Electronic Survey," *Midwifery* 79 (Dec. 2019): 102535. doi: 10.1016/j.midw.2019.102535.

5. P. Kranke, T. Frambach, P. Schelling, J. Wirbelauer, C. Schaefer, and U. Stamer, "Anaesthesia and Breast-Feeding: Should Breast-Feeding Be Discouraged?" *Anaesthesiologie Intensivmedizen Notfallmedizen Schmerztherapie* 46, no. 5 (May 2011): 304–11. doi: 10 .1055/s-0031-1277971.

CHAPTER 6

1. K. Uvnäs-Moberg, G. Marchini, and J. Winberg, "Plasma Cholecystokinin Concentrations After Breast Feeding in Healthy 4-Day-Old Infants," *Archives of Disease in Childhood* 68 (Jan. 1993): 46–48. doi: 10.1136/adc.68.1_spec_no.46.

CHAPTER 9

1. M. Wu, R. Chason, and M. Wong, "Raynaud's Phenomenon of the Nipple," *Obstetrics & Gynecology* 119, no. 2, pt. 2 (Feb. 2012): 447–49. doi: 10.1097/AOG.0b013e31822c9a73.

2. S. Watkins, S. Melter Broday, D. Zolnoun, and A. Stuebe. "Early Breastfeeding Experiences and Postpartum Depression," *Obstetrics & Gynecology* 118, no. 2, pt. 1 (Aug. 2011): 214–21.

3. J. Pawluski, M. Li, and J. Lonstein, "Serotonin and Motherhood: From Molecules to Mood," *Frontiers in Neuroendocrinology* 53 (Apr. 2019): 100742. doi: 10.1016/j.yfrne.2019.03.001.

CHAPTER 10

1. S. Schlatter, W. Schupp, J. Otten, S. Harnisch, M. Kunze, D. Stavropoulou, and R. Hentschel, "The Role of Tongue-Tie in Breastfeeding Problems—A Prospective Observational Study," *Acta Paediatrica* 108, no. 12 (Dec. 2019): 2214–21. doi: 10.1111/apa.14924.

2. C. W. Genna and E. V. Coryllos, "Breastfeeding and Tongue-Tie," *Journal of Human Lactation* 25, no. 1 (Feb. 2009): 111–12. doi: 10.1177/08903344090250011501.

3. B. A. Ghaheri, M. Cole, S. C. Fausel, M. Chuop, and J. C. Mace, "Breastfeeding Improvement Following Tongue-Tie and Lip-Tie Release: A Prospective Cohort Study," *Laryngoscope* 127, no. 5 (May 2017): 1217–23. doi: 10.1002/lary.26306.

CHAPTER 11

1. D. T. Ramsay, L. R. Mitoulas, J. C. Kent, M. Larsson, and P. E. Hartmann, "The Use of Ultrasound to Characterize Milk Ejection in Women Using an Electric Breast Pump," *Journal of Human Lactation* 21, no. 4 (Nov. 2005): 421–28. doi: 10.1177/08903344052 80878.

2. D. K. Prime, D. T. Geddes, D. L. Spatz, M. Robert, N. J. Trengove, and P. E. Hartmann, "Using Milk Flow Rate to Investigate Milk Ejection in the Left and Right Breasts During Simultaneous Breast Expression in Women," *International Breastfeeding Journal* 4, no. 10 (Oct. 2009). doi: 10.1186/1746-4358-4-10.

3. D. K. Prime, C. P. Garbin, P. E. Hartmann, and J. C. Kent, "Simultaneous Breast Expression in Breastfeeding Women Is More Efficacious than Sequential Breast Expression," *Breastfeeding Medicine* 7, no. 6 (Dec. 2012): 442–47. doi: 10.1089/bfm.2011.0139.

4. A. M. Demir, Z. Kuloglu, M. Berberoglu, and A. Kansu, "Euprolactinemic Galactorrhea Secondary to Domperidone Treatment," *Journal of Pediatric Endocrinology and Metabolism* 28, nos. 7–8 (July 2015): 955–56. doi: 10.1515/jpem-2014-0118.

5. P. J. Buffery and R. M. Strother, "Domperidone Safety: A Mini-Review of the Science of QT Prolongation and Clinical Implications of Recent Global Regulatory Recommendations," *New Zealand Medical Journal* 128, no. 1416 (June 2015): 66–74.

6. R. J. Osborne, M. L. Slevin, R. W. Hunter, and J. Hamer, "Cardiac Arrhythmias During Cytotoxic Chemotherapy: Role of Domperidone," *Human Toxicology* 4, no. 6 (Nov. 1985): 617–26. doi: 10 .1177/096032718500400608.

7. J. Q. Chen, H. Mori, R. D. Cardiff, J. F. Trott, R. C. Hovey, N. E. Hubbard, J. A. Engelberg, C. G. Tepper, B. J. Willis, I. H. Khan, R. K. Ravindran, S. R. Chan, R. D. Schreiber, and A. D. Borowsky, "Abnormal Mammary Development in 129:STAT1-Null Mice Is Stroma-Dependent," *PLoS One* 10, no. 6 (June 2015): e0129895. doi: 10.1371/journal.pone.0129895.

8. A. Zapantis, J. Steinberg, and L. Schilit, "Use of Herbals as Galactagogues," *Journal of Pharmacy Practrice,* 25, no. 2 (Apr. 2012): 222–31. doi: 10.1177/0897190011431636.

9. M. Mortel and S. Mehta, "Systematic Review of the Efficacy of Herbal Galactogogues," *Journal of Human Lactation* 29, no. 2 (May 2013): 154–62. doi: 10.1177/0890334413477243.

10. N. Bernard, H. Jantzem, M. Becker, C. Pecriaux, A. Bénard-Laribière, J. L. Montastruc, J. Descotes, T. Vial / French Network of Regional Pharmacovigilance Centres, "Severe Adverse Effects of Bromocriptine in Lactation Inhibition: A Pharmacovigilance Survey," *British Journal of Obstetrics and Gynaecology* 122, no. 9 (Aug. 2015): 1244–51. doi: 10.1111/1471-0528.13352.

CHAPTER 13

1. S. H. Jaafar, S. Jahanfar, M. Angolkar, and J. J. Ho, "Pacifier Use Versus No Pacifier Use in Breastfeeding Term Infants for Increasing Duration of Breastfeeding," *Cochrane Database of Systematic Reviews* 3 (Mar. 2011): CD007202. doi: 10.1002/14651858.CD 007202.pub2.

2. L. R. Kair, D. Kenron, K. Etheredge, A. C. Jaffe, and C. A. Phillipi, "Pacifier Restriction and Exclusive Breastfeeding," *Pediatrics* 131, no. 4 (Apr. 2013): e1101-17. doi: 10.1542/peds.2012-2203.

INDEX

Note: Page numbers in *italics* refer to figures.